2025-2026
Skincare
Blueprint

The Complete Guide to Clear, Radiant, and Ageless Skin for All Skin Types

Whitney F. Bowe

Copyright

2025–2026 Skincare Blueprint

Copyright © 2025 Whitney F. Bowe

All rights reserved. No part of this publication may be reproduced or transmitted in any form or by any means, electronic or mechanical, including photocopying, recording, or by any information storage and retrieval system, without permission in writing from the publisher.

While the advice and information in this book are believed to be true and accurate at the date of publication, neither the author, editors, nor the publisher can accept any legal responsibility for any errors or omissions that may be made. The publisher makes no warranty, express or implied, with respect to the material contained herein.

Disclaimer

This book is intended to provide general information on skincare and related topics. It is sold with the understanding that the author and publisher are not engaged in rendering medical, dermatological, or other professional services. If medical or dermatological advice or assistance is required, the services of a qualified health care provider should be sought.

Printed on acid-free paper..

Contents

Copyright i
Introduction 1
Chapter One 3
The Science of Skin 3
More Than Just a Barrier 6
Chapter Two 9
Skin Types and How to Identify Yours 9
Oily Skin 9
Dry skin 10
Combination Skin 11
Normal skin 12
Sensitive skin 12
Hormonal Skin 13
Identifying Your Skin Type 14
Caring for Your Skin Type 16
Managing Different the Skin Types 18
How Our Skin Change Over Time 19
Common Skin Concerns 20
Chapter Three 35
Building Your Skincare Routine 35
Morning Skincare Routine 35
Evening Skincare rituals 37
Cleansing 37
Types of Cleanser for different skins 39

Best cleanser active ingredients for different skins 41

Steps for Cleansing 44

Exfoliating, Why and How to Do It Safely 47

Exfoliating by Skin Type 49

Exfoliation by Body Part 50

Avoiding Skin Injury During Exfoliating 51

Moisturizing by Skin Type 52

Key ingredients to search for in moisturizers 54

Sunscreen 54

Benefits of Sunscreen 55

Types of Sun Screens and Their Protective Level 56

Anti-Aging Routine 58

Chapter Four 60

Enhancing Your Routine 60

Facial Oils 61

Face Oil Based On Skin Types 61

Tips to Get the Most from Face Oils 65

Correct Application of Facial Oil and Benefits 66

Face Mask: Indulgence or Necessity? 67

Types of Face Masks 67

Face Mask Benefits and How to Use its 68

Eye Creams: Targeting the Delicate Eye Area 70

Benefit of Eye Creams and How to Apply them 70

Types of Eye Creams 71

Key Difference between Morning vs. Nighttime Routines ... 72

Chapter Five **74**
Seasonal Adjustments to Your Routine **74**
Summer Skincare Routine 76
Transitioning Between Seasons 78

Chapter Six **81**
Skincare Active Ingredients and their functions **81**

Chapter Seven **90**
Natural and Synthetic Ingredients **90**
Understanding Synthetic Skincare Ingredients 91

Chapter Eight **94**
Ingredients to Avoid **94**
Fragrance: Yay or Nay? 96
Harsh Preservatives and Parabens 98
Types of Parabens 99
Why you should Avoid Parabens based products 99
Skincare During Pregnancy 100

Chapter Nine **102**
Age-based Skincare Routine **102**
Skincare for Teens 102
Building a Simple, Effective Routine 103
Morning Skincare Routine 103
Evening Skincare Routine 105
Additional Tips and Considerations 107
Skincare in your 20s 108
Requirement to maintain a healthy skin in my twenties (20s) 109

Skincare Routine in my Twenties (20s) 110
Anti-aging Products in my Twenties (20s) 111
Components of Skincare Product in your 20s 111
Skincare routine for different skin types in your 20s 111
Preventative Care 112
Managing Acne in your 20s 113
Effective Skincare Routine for Hormonal Acne 115

Chapter Ten 117
Skincare in Your 30s 117
Maintaining a Healthy Glow 118

Chapter Eleven 123
Skincare in Your 40s and Beyond 123
Primary causes of loss of elasticity 123
Areas susceptible to sagging 124
Techniques for restoring firmness 124
Managing Age Spots and Wrinkles 125

Chapter Twelve 128
Advanced Skincare 128
Chemical Peels 130
Microdermabrasion 131
Laser Treatments 131
Botox and Fillers 133

Chapter Thirteen 136
DIY Treatments at Home 136
Types of Do-it-yourself Chemical Peels 136

Microneedling Devices 138
LED Light Therapy 140
Red LED Light Therapy 141
Blue LED light therapy 142
Green LED Light Therapy 143
Yellow LED Light Therapy 143
White LED Light Therapy 144
When not to Use LED Light Therapy 145

Chapter Fourteen 147
Some Skincare Myths 147

Chapter Fifteen 150
Lifestyle and Skincare... 150
The Importance of Hydration in Skin Health 151
Foods for Healthy Skin...152
Stress and Sleep 153
Tips for Better Sleep and Skin Recovery 154
Exercise and Skin Health 158
Preventing Post-Workout Breakouts..159

Chapter Sixteen.. 162
Skincare on a Budget and When to Splurge 162
Affordable Drugstore Brands 163
Multi-Use Products 164
When to Splurge 164

Chapter Seventeen 166
Simplifying Your Routine... 166

The Rise of Minimal Skincare 166
Benefits of Minimalist Skincare Routines 168
Chapter Eighteen **170**
Skincare Routine for Men **170**
Common Skincare Issues for Men 170
Addressing Unique Skin Concerns 171
Simplify the Routine 174
Final Thoughts **175**
Staying Consistent for Long-Term Results 177
Where to Find Reliable Skincare Resources 178
Appendices 182
Glossary of Skincare Terms 182
SKIN TERMS/CONCERNS **184**
Product Recommendations by Category 191
Frequently Asked Skincare Questions and Answers 193
About the Author 207

Introduction

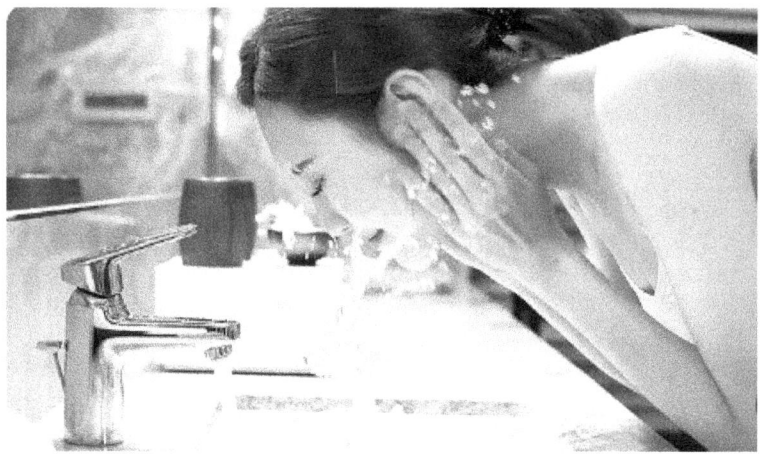

Taking care of the skin plays a key role in staying clean and avoiding infections. This usually starts with something as simple as washing with regular or antiseptic soap. Some also use alcohol-based solutions and lotions to help keep the skin healthy. Skin care routines can involve different steps to keep the skin in good shape, improve how it looks, and deal with various skin problems. Eating well, staying out of the sun for too long, and using moisturizers the right way all help protect the skin. Some routines focus more on improving appearance. These may include the use of makeup, retinol products, injections, chemical treatments, scrubs, laser treatments, microdermabrasion, fillers, or ultrasound-based procedures.

People often include skin care in their everyday habits, especially when managing dryness, irritation, or preventing damage. It also plays a role in keeping the face fresh and supporting skin repair. Products used at home can include both cosmetic and medicinal creams or serums. More people today are taking better care of themselves, and skin care has become a regular part of that. A well-kept routine helps your skin stay clear and smooth, even with exposure to dirt or harsh weather. It helps clean out clogged pores, limits breakouts, reduces dark spots from the sun, and leaves the skin looking soft and healthy.

Chapter One

The Science of Skin

Knowing your skin type is the first step in choosing the right products and building a routine that actually works for you. Whether your skin leans toward dry, oily, normal, combination, or sensitive, using products that match your needs can make a real difference. When your routine suits your skin, the result is often a smooth, clear, and radiant appearance—what many refer to as "glass skin." More than just looking good, this can also help you feel more relaxed and confident. That's why it's worth taking the time to understand how your skin behaves and what it needs to stay in good shape.

Your skin type is shaped by how your skin responds to everyday factors like weather, personal care products, and changes in hormones. It often comes down to how much oil your skin makes, how much water it holds, and how it reacts to different ingredients and conditions. The usual categories are dry, oily, combination, normal, and sensitive, and each one has its own set of needs. Still, it's common for someone to have a mix—for example, skin that feels both dry and easily irritated, or skin that changes with the seasons.

Having a regular routine helps your skin stay in good condition, but no single approach works for everyone. That's why knowing your skin type matters. Once you understand what kind of skin you have, you can use that information to choose products that support it instead of working against it. Think of it as giving your skin what it naturally responds to, not trying to change it completely.

The American Academy of Dermatology has outlined five main skin types—dry, oily, combination, normal, and sensitive. Each comes with its own traits and care approach, which affect how your skin feels and looks. So when you're putting together a routine, it's best to begin by figuring out where your skin fits. That way, you can select products that are made for your specific needs and avoid trial-and-error that might lead to irritation or dullness. The right mix can help reduce common problems like breakouts, dryness, or uneven tone, while keeping your skin looking fresh and well-balanced.

If you're unsure what your skin type is, don't worry—you're not alone. Most people are still figuring it out. We'll go through the basics of how to spot the different types and what sets them apart. There's no universal solution to glowing skin, but once you know your type, it becomes much easier to build a routine that gives real results.

Your skin type is mostly determined by the amount of oil your skin produces. This is often linked to your genes, but other things like hormone shifts, getting older, changes in weather, and stress levels can also play a role. Research has shown that your skin type can shift over time. For example, some people may find their skin becomes less oily as they get older or depending on humidity levels.

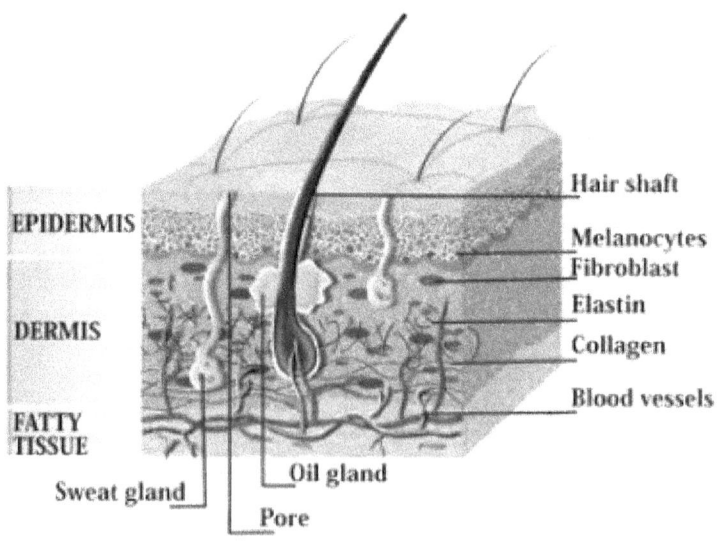

The basics of skin include how it is built, what it does, and the best ways to care for it. Skin is the body's largest organ and is made up of different types of cells. It consists of three main layers: the epidermis, the dermis, and the hypodermis. The epidermis is the outermost part, responsible for protecting the body and giving skin its color. Beneath that lies the dermis, which contains sweat glands, hair roots, nerve endings, and blood vessels. The deepest layer, the hypodermis, acts as a cushion and helps with insulation.

The skin plays several roles in keeping the body balanced and safe. It serves as a shield against harmful elements from the environment. It also helps regulate body temperature and allows us to feel sensations such as heat, cold, and pressure through nerve endings embedded in the layers. Looking after the skin involves a few daily steps. Washing helps remove dirt, oil, and dead skin cells. Moisturizing keeps the skin soft, smooth, and well-hydrated. Exfoliating clears out the pores and can improve how the skin feels and looks. Using sunscreen helps prevent damage caused by the sun and reduces the risk of early aging. Choosing the right products becomes much easier when you know your skin type, as this helps you care for it in a way that suits its natural behavior.

The epidermis is the outermost part of your skin—the layer you can see and touch. It's made up of cells built with a protein called keratin, which, along with other proteins, holds the cells together to form this protective surface. One of its main jobs is to act as a shield, keeping out harmful microorganisms and preventing infections. It also helps block the effects of weather, whether it's sun, rain, or wind. This layer is always at work, constantly creating new skin cells to replace the ones that are shed—about 40,000 every day. In roughly a month, you get a full layer of new skin. The epidermis also supports the body's defense system through cells called Langerhans cells, which help guard against germs and other threats.

Another role of the epidermis is providing pigment. It contains melanin, the substance that gives your skin its tone. The amount of melanin you produce determines the color of your skin, hair, and eyes. People with higher melanin levels often have darker skin and may tan more easily.

Beneath this is the dermis, which makes up most of your skin's thickness. This layer is packed with collagen and elastin—proteins that give skin strength and the ability to stretch and return to shape. The dermis also supports hair growth, with hair roots embedded deep within it. This layer is full of sensory nerves that help you notice changes around you. It picks up sensations like heat, touch, pain, and itchiness. Oil glands found here help keep your skin soft and prevent it from soaking up too much water when you're in the rain or swimming. The sweat glands also live here, producing sweat that helps cool your body down when it's warm. Finally, the dermis contains blood vessels that bring oxygen and nutrients to the skin's surface, keeping the outer layer in good condition. Below the dermis lies the hypodermis—the bottom layer of the skin. This layer is made up mostly of fat. It serves as a cushion, helping to protect muscles and bones from impact. It also holds tissue that connects the skin to muscles and bones underneath.

The nerves and blood vessels that begin in the dermis grow larger as they reach the hypodermis. From here, they spread out and link to other areas of the body. This layer also plays a part in managing your body temperature. The fat it holds helps prevent you from getting too cold or too hot, acting as natural insulation.

More Than Just a Barrier

Seeing the skin as nothing more than a shield between the body and the outside world doesn't truly reflect everything it does. While protecting against infection and keeping fluids in are essential tasks, the skin performs many other roles that work closely with other systems in the body. Special immune cells such as lymphocytes and dendritic cells help manage defense responses. The skin also plays a part in regulating body heat through its network of small blood vessels and sweat glands, assisted by the nervous system, which adjusts blood flow and sweating depending on the situation. Because the entire surface is exposed to the environment, it also helps with the transfer of heat. The skin is also packed with nerve endings that allow it to collect and send detailed messages to the brain. These signals come from specialized structures within the skin that are made to detect things like pressure, temperature, and texture. This means the skin is more than a physical cover—it's a living part of the body that not only protects but also feels, reacts, and takes part in chemical processes. Learning more about these roles helps caregivers understand why skin care matters and why wounds can affect more than just the surface. The skin keeps essential nutrients and chemicals inside the body while also standing guard against harmful substances and ultraviolet rays from sunlight. At the same time, things like skin tone, folds, and surface detail are part of what makes each person unique.

When the skin's normal function is disrupted or its appearance changes, it can affect both body and mind. Some skin issues stay local, but others might point to a condition affecting deeper systems. That's why medical professionals often need to look beyond the skin when dealing with visible symptoms. They may need to request blood work or other tests to check if something more is going on. The skin carries out a number of roles. One of the most important is protection. It guards against infections, toxins, and physical injury. The outer layer helps block viruses, bacteria, and anything else that may cause harm. It also stops damage from UV rays and creates a surface that discourages the growth of harmful germs.

Another key function is absorption. Some substances, including ingredients in creams or ointments, can pass through the skin and reach affected areas. This makes it easier to apply treatments directly where they're needed. The skin also helps balance body temperature. It does this by producing sweat and adjusting how much blood flows near the surface. When it's warm, sweating helps cool the body and blood vessels widen to let off heat. In colder conditions, the vessels narrow to hold in warmth.

Through its nerve endings, the skin gives us the sense of touch. It lets us feel pressure, temperature, pain, and soft contact, helping us avoid harm and interact with the world. Specific receptors in the skin—such as those for light touch, pain, and vibrations—make this possible. Another important role involves sunlight. When exposed to UV rays, the skin produces vitamin D, which supports healthy bones and helps the immune system. It also helps convert certain chemicals into active substances like hormones, which take part in many body functions.

Chapter Two

Skin Types and How to Identify Yours

Skin types can vary from person to person. Some people deal with excess oil, while others may notice dryness or a mix of both. There are also those whose skin reacts easily to products or changes in the environment. The most common skin types include oily, dry, combination, normal, sensitive, and those affected by hormonal changes.

Curious about which one applies to you? Paying attention to how your skin feels and behaves throughout the day can help you figure it out. Whether it stays balanced, gets shiny, feels tight, shows signs of irritation, or shifts during different times of the month, these signs can give you a better idea of how your skin naturally responds. Understanding these patterns is the first step to choosing the kind of care that suits you best.

Oily Skin

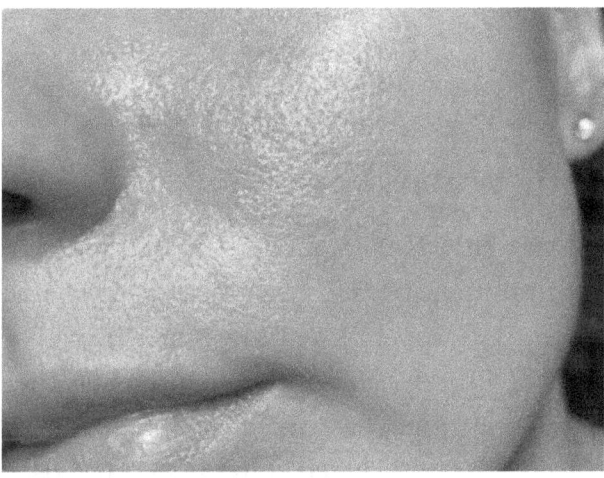

A skin is said to be Oily when the sebaceous glands produce more sebum than your body needs. This can be linked to your genes, changes in hormones, warmer weather, or even emotional stress. When there's too much oil, your face might appear shiny or greasy, especially in areas like the forehead, nose, and chin—commonly known as the T-zone.

This extra oil can also clog pores, which may lead to larger pore size, blackheads, or different types of breakouts. While it can be frustrating to manage, there are some upsides. According to the American Academy of Dermatology, people with oily skin might notice fewer lines and wrinkles as they age, thanks to the skin's natural moisture barrier.

Dry skin

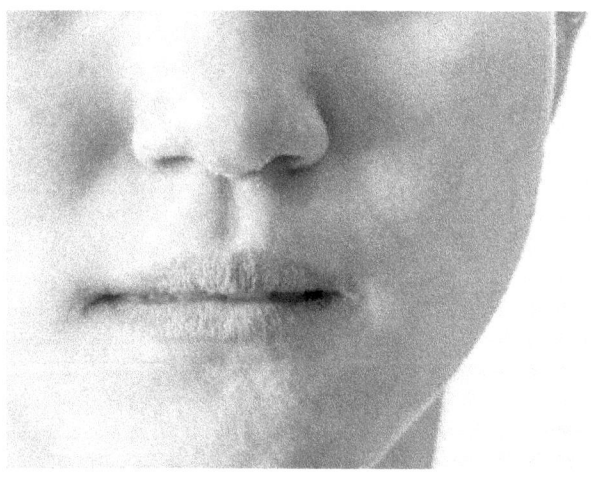

Dry skin produces far less natural oil compared to other skin types. These oils are important because they help keep the skin soft and prevent water from escaping. When there isn't enough oil, moisture tends to evaporate quickly, leaving the skin feeling rough, tight, or patchy. It might appear dull, flaky, or uneven in texture, and in some cases, it can feel itchy or irritated. Fine lines may also seem more noticeable due to the lack of hydration.

Several things can lead to dryness, with one of the main reasons being a damaged outer layer. This layer helps lock in moisture, but when it doesn't work well, water can escape more easily, leaving the skin dry and uncomfortable. Certain daily habits can make this worse—using products that strip away moisture or spending too much time in hot showers may cause the skin to lose even more hydration.

Combination Skin

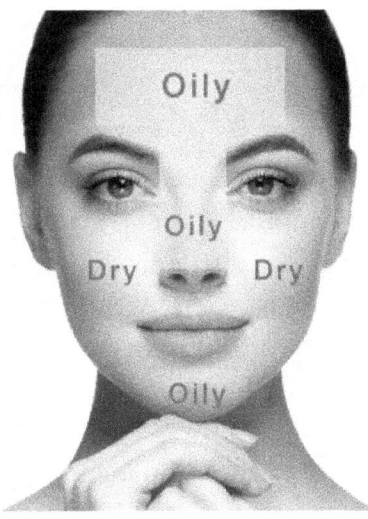

Combination skin means that some parts of your face are more oily, while others feel dry. In most cases, the forehead, nose, and chin—the area known as the T-zone—tend to be oilier, while the cheeks are often on the drier side. This skin type doesn't look the same for everyone. Some people may notice extra shine where their skin makes more oil, while others may deal with dryness that shows up as redness or rough spots. Depending on your natural skin tone, dry patches might even appear dull or grayish.

This skin type can also shift over time. It might feel different as the seasons change or react to things like stress or hormone changes.

Because of that, what works well for combination skin during one part of the year may need adjusting later on.

Normal skin

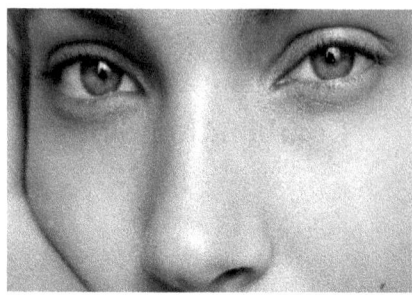

Normal skin means the skin is balanced, feeling neither too dry nor too oily. Unlike combination skin, people with this type don't usually deal with areas that shift between oiliness and dryness. Instead, their skin tends to feel even and comfortable all over.

This skin type often appears smooth and fresh, without signs of extra shine or dry patches. Pores are usually small and not very noticeable. Breakouts, redness, or other common issues are less frequent, and the skin doesn't react as easily to products or weather changes. Overall, it stays in a steady condition without needing much correction.

Sensitive skin

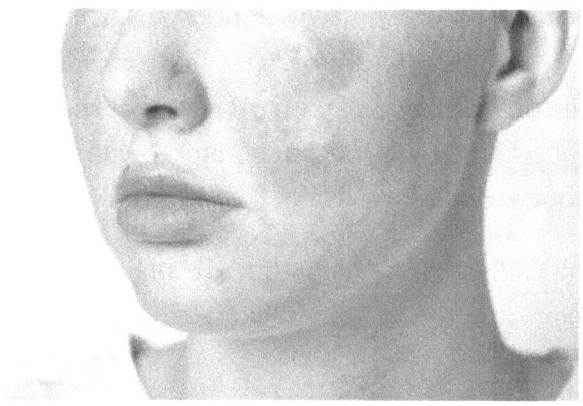

Sensitive skin is unique because it isn't defined by how much oil the skin produces. Instead, it refers to skin that reacts more easily than others. People with this skin type often notice discomfort when exposed to certain ingredients, like added fragrances, or when faced with environmental triggers such as air pollution or weather changes.

Reactions can show up as redness, stinging, burning, or a general feeling of irritation after using certain products. While it's seen as its own category, sensitivity can occur alongside oily, dry, combination, or even balanced skin. The exact reason why some people have sensitive skin isn't fully understood, though newer studies suggest it could be related to a weakened skin barrier that makes the skin less able to protect itself from outside elements.

Hormonal Skin

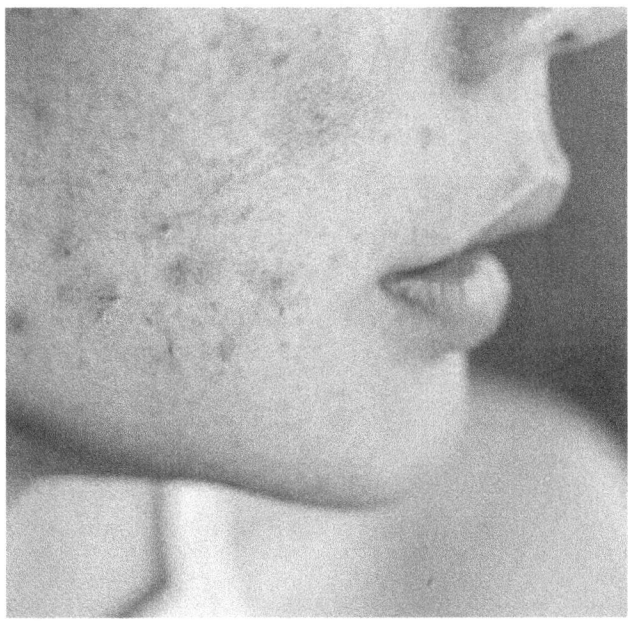

Hormonal skin refers to skin that changes in response to hormone levels. These shifts often happen around life stages such as menstruation, pregnancy, or menopause. During these times, the skin may produce more oil than usual, leading to breakouts—often in the T-zone, which includes the forehead, nose, and chin. At the same time, other parts of the face might feel dry or tight.

This skin type may also come with deeper breakouts that appear regularly, especially at certain points in a cycle. These changes are common, but they can be frustrating. If you notice patterns like this—oilier areas showing up on skin that's normally dry or breakouts appearing month after month—it may be worth speaking with a dermatologist. They can help confirm the cause and suggest the right steps to take. Hormonal skin often shows itself through a few common signs. One of the most noticeable is recurring breakouts that appear in the same areas—especially around the chin and jawline—just before your menstrual cycle begins.

You might also notice a greasy look across your forehead, nose, and chin, while the cheeks remain dry or feel tight. This mix of oily and dry areas is another common feature. Breakouts can sometimes include deep, painful pimples that seem to come out of nowhere. These tend to be larger and sit deeper under the skin. Changes in how your skin feels are also common. Some parts may feel smooth, while others feel rough or bumpy, making the surface look uneven. Another sign is how your skin shifts over the course of your cycle—some days it may look balanced, and on others, it may seem oilier or more textured than usual. These ups and downs often point to hormonal changes at work.

Identifying Your Skin Type

There are a few simple ways you can check your skin type at home. These methods can give you a clearer idea of how your skin behaves and what kind of care it might need. One common method is often called the "watch and wait" or "bare-faced" approach. You start by washing your face with a mild cleanser, then gently pat it dry. Without applying anything else, wait for about 30 minutes and look at your skin in the mirror. If your face appears shiny everywhere, that's a sign of oily skin. If your skin feels tight, rough, or shows flaking, it's likely dry. Shine only in the forehead, nose, and chin points to combination skin, while skin that feels balanced without dryness or oil suggests a normal skin type.

Another simple way to figure it out is by using blotting papers. After cleansing and drying your face, wait 30 minutes, then press a clean blotting sheet against different parts of your face. Hold the sheet up to the light. If you notice a lot of oil across all areas, you may have oily skin. Barely any oil suggests dryness. Oil only in the T-zone can mean combination skin, while a small amount in all areas likely points to normal skin. You can also try the touch method. Clean your hands first, then use your fingertips to gently feel different areas of your face. If it feels slick or greasy—especially in the T-zone—you might have oily skin. If your skin feels rough, tight, or flaky, it's probably dry. When the forehead and nose feel oily but the cheeks seem dry or balanced, that's often combination skin. Sensitive skin might feel sore or show redness after even light contact, though not all sensitive skin reacts the same way. If your skin feels smooth without excess oil or dryness and shows no signs of redness or breakouts, you may have a normal skin type.

If you're still unsure or want more clarity, seeing a dermatologist or skin care professional can help. They can look at your skin closely, sometimes using special tools, and provide you with more specific guidance—especially if you're dealing with breakouts or other ongoing skin issues. Lastly, keep an eye on how your skin behaves throughout your monthly cycle. Changes in oil levels or breakouts at certain times may be linked to hormone shifts, and tracking these patterns can help you better understand what your skin needs.

Caring for Your Skin Type

Oily Skin: You can't completely get rid of oily skin, but you can manage it with the right care. A consistent routine can help reduce the shine and keep your face from looking greasy as the day goes on. So, what works best when dealing with oily skin? People with this skin type often stay away from products that include oil. Whether it's a cleanser or a moisturizer, choosing something labeled oil-free is usually a better option.

It's also a common mistake to think that oily skin doesn't need moisture. Even though your skin may produce more oil than others, it still needs hydration. Using a lightweight, oil-free moisturizer after washing your face can help maintain balance without clogging pores. Look for products that are gentle and made not to block the skin, especially if you're trying to avoid breakouts.

Dry Skin: For those with dry skin, it's best to start your routine with a gentle cleanser that doesn't contain fragrance. Choosing products with ingredients like ceramides—which help support your skin's natural barrier—and hyaluronic acid—which helps hold onto moisture—can be especially helpful. Glycerin is another ingredient worth considering, as it also draws in hydration. Even with dry skin, washing your face twice a day is fine, but it's important to follow up with a moisturizer right after to replace any moisture that may have been lost. Go for creams instead of lotions, as thicker products tend to provide more relief for dryness. These richer options can help keep the skin feeling soft and prevent it from drying out as quickly.

Combination Skin: Whether your skin is oily, dry, or a mix of both, keeping it clean and moisturized is important. When applying moisturizer, it's helpful to pay extra attention to the parts of your face that feel drier. For example, if your cheeks tend to be dry, you can apply a bit more product there than on other areas. One way to care for skin that has both oily and dry spots is by using two different moisturizers. A cream-based option works well for areas that need more hydration, while a lighter, gel-based one is better for spots that feel greasy. At night, you might choose a gel moisturizer for your T-zone and a thicker cream for your cheeks and neck. The specific brand is up to you—what matters most is how your skin responds.

If you notice extra shine during the day, especially on your forehead or nose, blotting papers can help absorb the oil without disturbing the rest of your routine.

Normal Skin: Although normal skin doesn't usually come with many issues, it still needs daily care to stay in good shape. A simple routine that keeps the skin hydrated while supporting its natural barrier is often enough. Even if your skin feels balanced, using a good moisturizer is still important. Products with ingredients like ceramides and hyaluronic acid can help lock in water and keep the skin feeling soft after cleansing. Just because your skin doesn't feel dry or oily doesn't mean you should skip this step. No matter your skin type—whether it's normal, oily, dry, sensitive, or a mix—it's still possible to experience breakouts. That's why it's a good idea to choose products that won't block your pores. Using non-comedogenic skincare and makeup can help reduce the chance of unexpected blemishes, even if your skin usually behaves well.

Sensitive Skin: If your skin reacts easily or often feels irritated, it's a good idea to meet with a board-certified dermatologist to find out what might be causing the problem. They can help you put together a daily routine that's better suited for skin that needs a gentle touch. This includes recommending mild cleansers, moisturizers, sunscreens, and other products that won't trigger discomfort.

They may also guide you on how to adjust parts of your environment—like household products or habits—to avoid contact with things that might be making your skin react. People with sensitive skin should stay away from anything overly harsh or drying, including products with added fragrance. Brands like CeraVe suggest keeping it simple with products made to comfort and support sensitive skin. Some examples include a gentle hydrating facial cleanser, a moisturizing serum with hyaluronic acid, and a mineral-based sunscreen with SPF 30 that also includes a light tint.

Managing Different the Skin Types

No matter what kind of skin you have, taking care of it the right way helps it stay clear, smooth, and fresh-looking. Below are some simple ways to care for different skin types. For oily skin, washing your face twice daily can help reduce extra oil and keep pores from becoming clogged. Adding exfoliation a few times a week helps clear away dirt and old skin cells. Choose moisturizers and sunscreens that are oil-free and won't block pores. During the day, using blotting sheets or products made to reduce shine can help your skin stay balanced.

If you have dry skin, it's important to keep it hydrated. Use creamy cleansers that clean without removing your skin's natural oils. Drinking enough water daily also supports hydration from within. With combination skin, different areas may need different care. A mild cleanser that balances the skin works well across the whole face. You can use richer products on dry spots and lighter ones on oily areas. Exfoliating once or twice a week helps remove buildup but avoid scrubbing too hard on the dry zones.

Those with sensitive skin should always test new products on a small patch before full use. Look for gentle, fragrance-free options made for sensitive skin. A shorter routine with calming ingredients is best to avoid triggering reactions. If your skin is well-balanced, you still need to maintain it. Use a gentle cleanser morning and night. A weekly exfoliation can help remove buildup. Wearing sunscreen daily protects your skin from sun damage, and staying away from harsh ingredients helps keep your skin steady.

For hormonal skin, cleansing with a soft touch helps remove oil without stressing the skin. You might find it helpful to use products with ingredients like salicylic acid or benzoyl peroxide to target breakouts, while hyaluronic acid can help keep dry areas comfortable. A steady routine, along with good rest, healthy meals, and managing stress, can make a difference. If the skin continues to act up, checking in with a doctor may help uncover any hormone-related causes.

How Our Skin Change Over Time

As you get older, your skin goes through a number of changes. You may notice that it becomes thinner, less firm, and not as smooth as it used to be. The top layer starts to lose some of its fullness and color, and the skin doesn't bounce back the way it once did. Over time, blood vessels beneath the skin can become more fragile, which means bruises might appear more easily. Sweat and oil production may also slow down with age. This can lead to skin that feels drier than before. Several factors play a role in how skin changes over the years. One of them is the natural loss of certain fibers in the skin—such as elastin and collagen—which help keep it firm and flexible. Without these, the skin begins to wrinkle and feel more fragile.

Hormonal shifts, such as those during menopause, can also lead to drier and thinner skin. Long-term health conditions that often affect older adults, such as diabetes, heart problems, or kidney issues, may also influence the way the skin looks and feels. Another major factor in skin aging is sun exposure. The sun gives off ultraviolet (UV) rays that can harm skin cells. While this may first appear as a sunburn, the damage builds up over time. As the years pass, that buildup can change the texture of your skin, bring on early signs of aging, and increase the chance of certain skin conditions—including skin cancer.

Common Skin Concerns

Acne and Breakouts: Acne is a condition where the pores of the skin become blocked by oil, dead skin, and bacteria. This leads to the development of blackheads, whiteheads, pimples, or cysts. When several blemishes show up around the same time, it is often called a breakout. While acne is most common during the teenage years and early adulthood, some persons continue to experience it later in life.

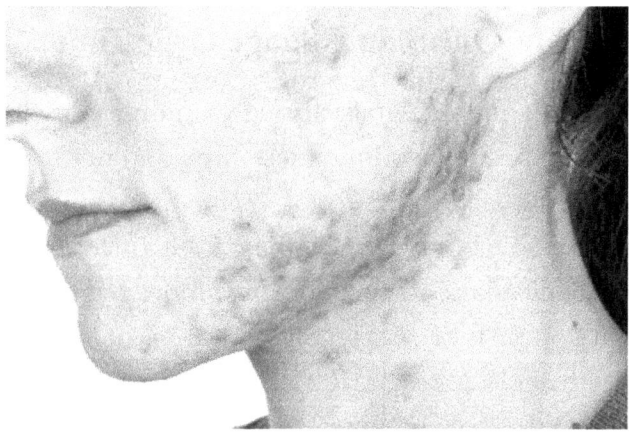

The main reason acne develops is due to clogged pores. These clogs can appear as different types of spots—some filled with pus and painful, others small and discolored. The term often used by doctors for acne is acne vulgaris. There are a few kinds of acne, each with unique traits. Cystic acne causes larger, painful lumps under the skin that often leave marks. Fungal acne, also known as pityrosporum folliculitis, is due to yeast building up in the hair follicles and often feels itchy. Hormonal acne appears when hormones increase oil production and block pores. Nodular acne involves both visible breakouts and deep, sore bumps under the skin. Acne can affect almost anyone, regardless of age. It's more common during times when hormones shift, like puberty, but adults—especially women—can also be affected. If others in your family have experienced acne, you might be more likely to have it too. This condition often appears on areas with many oil glands. Common places include the face, forehead, shoulders, chest, and upper back.

Some signs of acne include whiteheads and blackheads, which are blocked pores with either a light or dark surface. Papules are small, discolored bumps that may be red or darker than your skin tone. Pustules are pimples filled with pus. Nodules and cysts form deeper under the skin and are usually painful to the touch. The cause of acne starts with hair follicles becoming blocked. Each hair on your body grows from a follicle connected to glands that produce sebum, a natural oil that protects the skin. When excess oil, bacteria, or old skin cells build up inside the follicle, a blockage forms. This causes swelling, discomfort, and changes in skin color around the clogged pore. Doctors group acne into four stages depending on how serious it is. The first stage involves mostly blackheads and whiteheads with a few inflamed spots. The second includes more red or pus-filled pimples, mostly on the face. In stage three, the acne is more widespread and includes deeper bumps. The fourth and most severe stage involves many painful, inflamed nodules and cysts.

Treatment often depends on how mild or severe the acne is. For minor breakouts, store-bought creams, cleansers, and spot treatments are commonly used. Ingredients like benzoyl peroxide can dry up pimples and fight bacteria. Salicylic acid helps remove buildup and keep pores clear. For cases that don't improve with these products, it's a good idea to see a dermatologist. They might suggest stronger options, such as prescription creams or oral medications. These may include higher-strength benzoyl peroxide, antibiotics like erythromycin or clindamycin, or retinoids such as retinol. In some situations, birth control pills or other hormonal treatments might be used, especially if hormone shifts are part of the cause. Antibiotics are usually used for short periods to lower the risk of resistance.

In more serious cases, your doctor might combine different treatments. This could include oral antibiotics, topical retinoids, and creams. In some cases, a medication known as isotretinoin (often called Accutane) is prescribed. This vitamin A-based drug is known to help with severe acne, though it can have strong side effects, so it's only recommended when other treatments don't work. There are also in-office options available. These include procedures to improve the skin's texture and manage oil production. Photodynamic therapy uses special light and medication to reduce bacteria and oil buildup. Other laser-based methods can also target problem areas and marks. Dermabrasion uses a rotating brush to remove the surface layer of the skin, while microdermabrasion is a gentler version of this. Chemical peels remove the uppermost layer of the skin to bring out fresher skin underneath. Cortisone shots are sometimes used to reduce swelling in painful cysts and are often combined with other treatments.

Even when using acne treatments, breakouts can still happen. Acne can be triggered by different things in different people. However, there are steps you can take at home to support your skin while you're undergoing treatment. Keeping your face clean is important. Wash gently up to twice a day and after sweating, using a non-abrasive cleanser. Always use your fingers instead of rough tools like washcloths or sponges.

Pick products carefully. Choose gentle ones that don't contain alcohol or other ingredients that might cause dryness or irritation. Avoid toners, astringents, and harsh exfoliants if your skin is already reacting. Wash your hair regularly, especially if it tends to get oily. Hair oil can transfer to your forehead and contribute to breakouts. Stick to your treatment routine without switching products too often. Jumping from one product to another can irritate the skin and lead to more breakouts. Give your treatment time to work—some results may take a few weeks to appear. Try not to touch your face throughout the day. Picking or squeezing pimples can delay healing and may leave marks or discoloration behind.

Stay out of the sun and away from tanning beds. Tanning damages the skin and increases the risk of other conditions. Some acne treatments make the skin more sensitive to sunlight, so protection is extra important. Wear clothing that shields the skin and apply a broad-spectrum sunscreen with SPF 30 or higher on exposed areas. Look for sunscreens labeled "non-comedogenic" to reduce the risk of clogged pores. Some sun-protective clothing also includes a UPF rating for added coverage.

Wrinkles and Fine Lines: Wrinkles and fine lines form as part of the natural aging process. Over time, the skin begins to lose firmness and bounce, which leads to folds and creases. These lines often start out faint and gradually become more visible. Wrinkles are most noticeable on areas that are exposed to the sun, such as the face, neck, hands, and arms. They may look like small grooves or lines in the skin, much like fabric that hasn't been smoothed out.

Several factors can lead to the development of wrinkles. One of the most common reasons is aging. As the years go by, skin cells divide at a slower rate, and the surface of the skin becomes thinner. From around the age of 30, the body starts losing a small percentage of collagen each year. Collagen plays a big role in keeping the skin firm and strong. Repeated facial movements, such as smiling, frowning, or squinting, also contribute to wrinkles over time. As the skin loses fat and bone support, and gravity pulls it downward, lines can become more permanent—especially between the brows and at the corners of the eyes.

Too much sun exposure also affects the skin. Ultraviolet rays break down collagen, making it harder for the skin to stay firm. As a result, lines may appear sooner than expected. Smoking has a similar effect, slowing down the body's ability to make collagen, which makes the skin more likely to wrinkle.

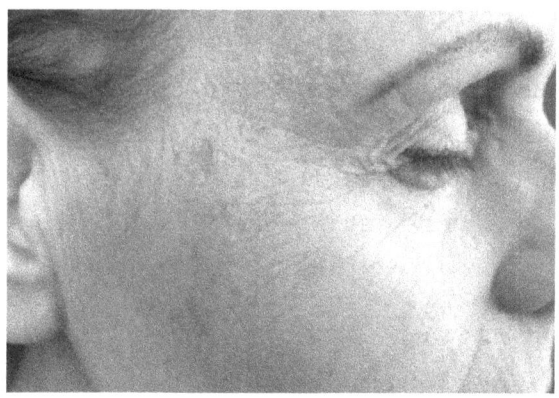

Wrinkles are a natural part of getting older, but there are treatments available for those who want to reduce their appearance. One common option is using products with retinoids, which are made from vitamin A. These ingredients help with texture, tone, and moisture, and can support the layers of the skin where collagen and elastin are found. You can find some versions of retinoids in over-the-counter creams, or a healthcare provider can suggest a stronger version suited to your needs.

Another method is micro-needling, which uses small needles to make tiny points in the skin. These tiny injuries prompt the body to heal by making new collagen and elastin, which can improve the look of fine lines. Microdermabrasion involves gently removing the top layer of skin, which can help with uneven tone, sun damage, and mild scars. A deeper version, called dermabrasion, goes further into the skin to smooth out rough texture and deeper lines. Chemical peels use a solution to take off the upper layer of skin, allowing smoother skin to grow in its place. These are used for lines, spots, and scarring. Laser resurfacing is another method used to target areas with wrinkles or past damage. A focused beam of light works on the layers of the skin to encourage new growth. This method is often used for fine lines under the eyes, around the mouth, and on the forehead. It can also help with acne scars. People with lighter skin tones may respond better to this method, as darker skin may develop changes in tone afterward.

Injections made from botulinum toxin, such as Botox®, help by relaxing the muscles that cause certain lines, especially those that appear when you frown or squint. These are often used between the eyebrows or near the eyes. For deeper lines that stay even when the face is resting, fillers may help. These are often used around the mouth, nose, and chin. One of the more common fillers is made from hyaluronic acid, which is a substance the body produces naturally. A more lasting option is a facelift. During this procedure, extra skin and fat are removed from the face and neck, and the layers underneath are tightened. This can reduce the look of lines and give the face a smoother shape. While wrinkles can't be completely avoided, there are simple habits that may help delay their appearance. These include using sunscreen every day, avoiding tanning beds, and keeping the skin moisturized. It's also helpful to wash your face after sweating heavily or wearing makeup for long periods.

Staying away from smoking and cutting down on alcohol can also make a difference. Drinking enough water and eating a balanced diet full of vitamins and nutrients can support overall skin health too.

Hyperpigmentation and Dark Spots: Hyperpigmentation, often referred to as dark spots, is a common skin concern caused by a variety of internal and environmental factors. While it can be upsetting for those affected, the good news is that it can be managed. The term describes areas of the skin that appear darker than the surrounding skin and may result from acne, sun exposure, or other conditions. Though it may stand out visually, hyperpigmentation is usually not harmful. These darker patches form when the skin produces extra melanin—the pigment responsible for the color of your skin, hair, and eyes. Melanin also helps protect the skin and eyes from harmful rays from the sun. This condition can occur in any skin tone, and it often appears as uneven patches or spots on the face or body.

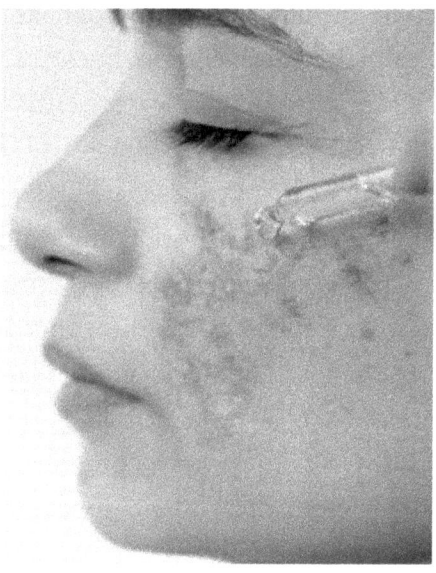

There are several types of hyperpigmentation. These include age spots (sometimes called sunspots or liver spots), melasma (often seen during pregnancy), and post-inflammatory dark marks that follow skin injuries or breakouts. Certain medications and health problems can also lead to this condition. Sun exposure is one of the most frequent triggers. Areas like the face, arms, and hands, which are exposed more often, are especially at risk. Hormonal changes, such as those during pregnancy or caused by birth control, can also play a role. Some medications, including anti-inflammatory drugs, chemotherapy treatments, anti-malarials, and anticonvulsants, may contribute to darkening of the skin.

Inflammation from conditions like eczema, psoriasis, or acne can leave behind dark spots after healing. Even a healed burn, insect bite, or scratch can result in lingering discoloration. Some cosmetic products may also irritate the skin and cause marks to form. Health conditions like diabetes may also affect the skin's appearance. For example, people with diabetes may notice dark patches on their shins or other parts of the body. These include conditions like diabetic dermopathy, acanthosis nigricans, necrobiosis lipoidica, and eruptive xanthomatosis—all of which can cause darker or raised spots on different areas of the skin. In rare cases, a new dark mark might point to a more serious issue such as skin cancer. Signs that could suggest melanoma include asymmetry, uneven borders, color changes, a spot larger than a quarter of an inch, or one that changes in size or appearance.

Managing hyperpigmentation depends on what's causing it. Some cases can be treated at home, while others may need attention from a dermatologist. Here are a few approaches that can help improve the look of dark spots: Brightening creams are widely used and can be effective, though the results may take some time. These creams often contain ingredients that help fade discoloration and encourage even skin tone. Some versions available by prescription work faster and contain stronger active agents. A product like Neutrogena Bright Boost Gel Cream contains Neoglucosamine, which promotes skin renewal and may reduce the look of uneven patches. It also helps prevent excess pigment from forming. Sunscreen versions of these products, such as Neutrogena® Bright Boost Gel Fluid SPF 30, can protect your skin while addressing discoloration. These types of products often include ingredients like vitamin C, vitamin E, and antioxidants to support overall skin health.

Chemical peels are another method. These can be done at home or in a professional setting and help remove the top layer of skin to reveal a smoother surface underneath. Because this process makes skin more sensitive to sunlight, it's important to use sun protection after treatment. Cryotherapy is a method where unwanted skin tissue is frozen and removed. It's often used to treat growths like warts but may also be recommended to target certain types of dark spots. Microdermabrasion is a gentle procedure that scrubs away the top layer of dead skin cells. It's helpful for treating uneven skin tone and sun damage and can be done at a clinic or skincare center.

Intense Pulsed Light (IPL) therapy uses light pulses to target areas with uneven tone, lines, or visible signs of aging. It's a non-surgical option that may help with hyperpigmentation among other concerns. If you're struggling with dark spots, know that you're not alone—people deal with this issue, and there are many ways to address it. Whether you use store-bought treatments or visit a skin care professional, improvements are possible. Daily sunscreen use and regular moisturizing can go a long way in preventing future discoloration and maintaining the results of your skincare efforts.

Eczema and Psoriasis: Eczema and psoriasis are both long-term skin conditions that can cause itching, redness, and irritation. While they may seem similar at first glance, they have their differences. Eczema tends to cause intense itching and appears as rough, bumpy rashes, often found in body creases like behind the knees or inside the elbows. Psoriasis, on the other hand, usually forms thick, scaly patches. Neither condition has a permanent solution, but both can be managed with consistent skin care.

Eczema is often triggered by things in the environment, such as allergens or irritants. The most common form is atopic dermatitis, and people from all backgrounds may experience it. In the U.S., research shows that eczema affects about 13% of Asian Americans and Pacific Islanders, 13% of Native Americans, 11% of white individuals, and 10% of Black or African American individuals. Eczema can make the skin appear cracked or dry. It may look red on light skin and more brown, gray, or purple on darker tones. Though it can't be erased completely, there are remedies that help ease discomfort.

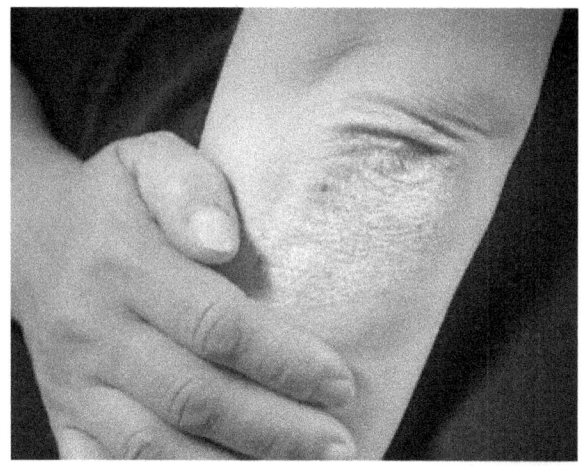

One well-known natural option is aloe vera gel. This soothing substance is taken from the aloe plant and has been used for thousands of years to calm the skin. Its properties can help prevent infections and support the healing process, especially when skin is cracked from dryness. Apple cider vinegar is another remedy used for skin care, though it should be used carefully. It may help with symptoms, but it needs to be diluted first to avoid damaging the skin. It can be used in damp cloth wraps or added to bathwater and is easy to find in grocery or health stores.

Some doctors also suggest adding a small amount of bleach to bathwater, which may help reduce bacteria on the skin. This is believed to help control flare-ups, especially those caused by bacteria like Staphylococcus aureus. A review in 2018 suggested that bleach baths might reduce the need for topical medicines, although other studies found no added benefit when compared to regular bathing. If discomfort or skin irritation occurs afterward, it's best to stop this method. Colloidal oatmeal is another gentle option. Made from finely ground oats, it has been shown to reduce itchiness, dryness, and rough patches. Mixing it into warm bathwater and soaking affected areas can calm the skin.

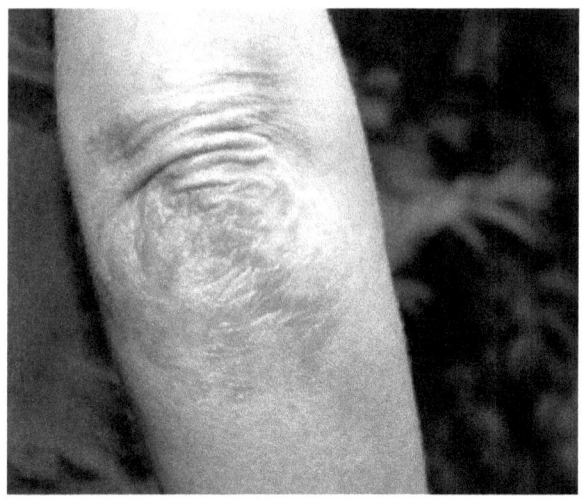

Bathing itself plays a role in managing eczema. Since the skin's outer layer often struggles to keep in moisture, regular baths can help—but only if done the right way. Using very hot or very cold water, or soaps that are too harsh, may make things worse. Moisturizing immediately after bathing is key. For young children and infants, bathing once or twice a week is often enough. Coconut oil may also be helpful. It contains fatty acids that moisturize the skin and may reduce inflammation. Using virgin coconut oil can help improve the skin's protective barrier and make it feel more comfortable. Honey has long been used to treat skin problems. It has both anti-inflammatory and germ-fighting properties. It may support healing and help the skin stay protected. Studies have looked at honey's ability to improve wounds, burns, and even some types of infections. Tea tree oil is a natural oil made from the leaves of the Melaleuca alternifolia tree. It's often used in skin care products and may help with eczema symptoms due to its anti-inflammatory and antibacterial effects. While more research is needed to understand its full impact on eczema, it remains a common choice in natural skin care. These remedies don't cure eczema, but brings comfort and reduce the frequency or intensity of symptoms. As with any skin care method, it's important to test a small amount first and speak to a healthcare provider if symptoms worsen.

Psoriasis is a long-term skin condition linked to the immune system. It causes itching, discomfort, and patches of thick, flaky skin. The most common type is plaque psoriasis, which forms raised areas covered in silvery scales. Although there is no permanent fix, different treatments can help ease the symptoms and improve comfort. Your doctor may suggest creams, medications, or other options to manage flare-ups and keep your skin as calm as possible. This condition leads to inflammation that affects the skin's surface. Patches can appear in various shapes and sizes and are often discolored and covered with scales. Because psoriasis tends to come and go, people may have long stretches without symptoms followed by periods of more active skin irritation.

There are several types of psoriasis, each with its own signs. Plaque psoriasis is the most widespread, affecting the majority of those with the condition. Inverse psoriasis develops in skin folds and appears as smooth patches without scales. Guttate psoriasis can follow a throat infection and often shows up as small, red spots with a flaky surface. Pustular psoriasis causes bumps filled with pus, and erythrodermic psoriasis affects large areas, leading to peeling and widespread discoloration. Sebopsoriasis appears around the face and scalp with greasy yellow flakes and is somewhat similar to seborrheic dermatitis. Nail psoriasis changes how the fingernails or toenails look, causing them to become discolored, brittle, or separated. Along with the appearance of plaques or rashes, people with psoriasis may also notice dryness, itching, cracking, or tenderness in the affected areas. In some cases, the nails may become chipped or damaged. Joint pain can also develop, which may be a sign of related arthritis. It's important not to scratch the affected skin, as this can open wounds and raise the risk of infection. Signs of an infection include pain, swelling, and fever. If any of these occur, it's important to seek medical attention right away.

Managing psoriasis often involves a mix of treatment approaches. Common options include steroid creams to calm the skin, moisturizers to reduce dryness, and prescription ointments that help slow down skin cell buildup. Some shampoos and body creams are made specifically for this condition. Products with vitamin D3 or vitamin A (retinoids) may also help with flare-ups. If the affected area is small, creams or ointments might be enough. For more widespread symptoms, or if joint pain is present, additional care may be needed. Your treatment plan will depend on how much of your skin is affected, where the rashes are located, your age, and your overall health. The goal is to keep the skin comfortable, reduce inflammation, and help prevent future outbreaks.

Enlarge Pores: Pores that appear larger than usual are often the result of skin producing too much oil or becoming clogged. This is common in people with oily skin or acne, where the sebaceous glands are more active. When excess oil builds up and blocks the opening of the pore, the walls can stretch, making the pores more visible. Other things that can make pores look bigger include aging, sun exposure, poor skincare habits, certain medications, and general skin imbalance caused by unsuitable products or health conditions.

One of the main approaches to dealing with noticeable pores is to focus on controlling oil production. Many acne treatments also help reduce pore size. In particular, some people have seen better skin texture through photodynamic therapy. Medicines such as oral isotretinoin, as well as topical versions like tretinoin and tazarotene, have shown promising results in improving how the skin looks by helping with oil regulation and refining pores. Glycolic acid peels—sometimes combined with vitamin C—are also known to improve the look of pores. Salicylic acid peels work well for acne-prone skin since they can reach into the pores and clean them out.

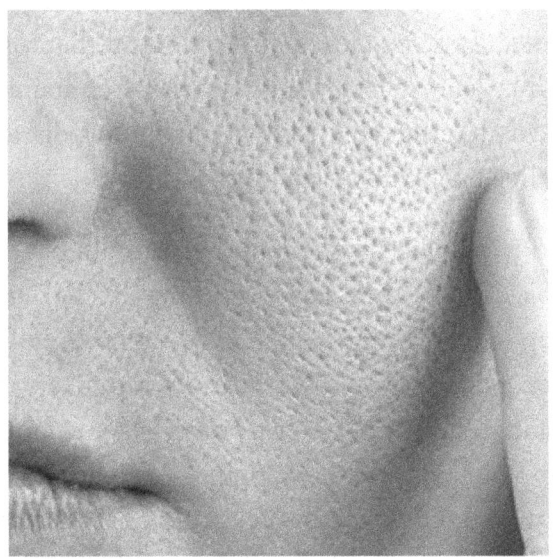

There has been some growing interest in the use of Botox for surface-level skin concerns. Instead of being injected into the muscles to control movement, it's used just below the skin's surface. This approach may influence the tiny muscles connected to oil glands, helping to prevent the pores from widening. Treatments like Aquagold fine touch demonstrate how this technique is applied. Another option that has gained popularity is a procedure known as Baby Fraxel. It uses a fractional laser to smooth the skin, stimulate collagen, and improve pore visibility. This device, also called the Smooth and Brilliant laser, works gently while delivering noticeable skin texture improvement. When used with a pigment-reducing serum like Permea, it can also help even out skin tone.

For those looking for ways to manage pores at home, there are several habits and products that may be helpful. Regular exfoliation is useful, but it's best to avoid harsh scrubs with rough particles that can damage the skin. If your current cleanser leaves your skin feeling clogged, consider switching to a foaming, water-based option. A mild salicylic acid moisturizer (around 1%) can be helpful; stronger versions might cause peeling. A quality cleansing brush like the Clarisonic can also make a difference. It helps clear out dirt and oil that might otherwise settle in the pores. Clay masks, especially those containing kaolin, can help keep the skin clear. It's best to avoid products with strong fragrances, as they can irritate sensitive skin.

Paying attention to your daily routine also matters. Eating enough fruits, vegetables, and fiber supports overall skin health. Always remove makeup before going to bed, and be mindful of what touches your skin. Even fabric softeners used on your sheets or pillowcases can leave behind residue that clogs pores—if you notice bumps or larger pores on your cheeks, try skipping softener and see if it helps. If you choose to extract clogged pores at home, take time to learn the correct method. Pressing too hard or using the wrong technique can push debris further into the skin and make the issue worse. With the right mix of care and consistency, it's possible to reduce the appearance of large pores and maintain a smoother, more balanced complexion.

Chapter Three

Building Your Skincare Routine

Clear, glowing skin is often the result of a consistent and thoughtful routine. With the right mindset and a little daily care, anyone can enjoy skin that looks refreshed and feels balanced. This guide walks you through an 8-step skincare routine that works well for all skin types, helping you maintain a healthy-looking complexion every day.

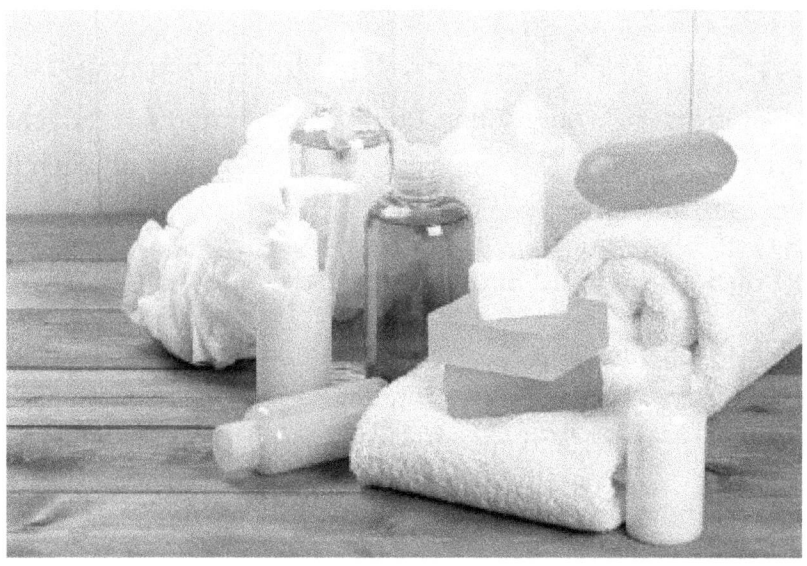

Morning Skincare Routine

Step One: Cleanse

Start your morning by washing your face to clear away any oil or buildup from the night. Choose a gentle cleanser that suits your skin type—whether it's dry, oily, or a mix of both—to avoid stripping away natural moisture. Keeping this first step simple and suitable for your skin helps lay the foundation for the rest of your routine.

Step two: Exfoliation (Remove dirt and dead cells by performing a thorough exfoliation).

Exfoliating your skin—whether using a gentle scrub or a chemical option—helps remove layers of dead cells that can cause blocked pores, uneven tone, breakouts, fine lines, and dark spots. Doing this no more than twice a week can help smooth your skin's surface, improve its clarity, and bring out a more refreshed, natural look.

Step three: Tone.

Toner plays a role in bringing balance to your skin's pH and getting it ready for the rest of your routine. For a fresh, comfortable feel, choose a formula made with gentle ingredients like rose water or witch hazel to help calm and refresh the surface.

Step Four: Antioxidant Serum

Including a vitamin C serum in your morning routine can help protect your skin from daily exposure to outdoor elements. It also supports a smoother appearance and encourages a natural, healthy-looking glow.

Step Five: moisturize.

Keep your skin soft and smooth by applying a light moisturizer that locks in moisture without making your face greasy. Choose one with ingredients like hyaluronic acid, which helps your skin hold onto water and stay comfortable throughout the day.

Step Six: Sunscreen.

Make sunscreen a part of your morning routine every day. Choose one with broad-spectrum protection and an SPF of 30 or higher to help protect your skin from sun damage and slow down signs of early aging.

Evening Skincare rituals

Step Seven: Double-cleanse

At night, start your routine by cleansing twice to make sure all traces of makeup, sunscreen, and daily buildup are fully removed. Use an oil-based cleanser first to break down any residue, followed by a water-based one to leave your skin feeling clean and refreshed.

Step 8: night cream or retinol

Complete your evening routine with a nourishing night cream or a product that contains retinol. Known for improving how the skin looks over time, retinol can help smooth out uneven texture and bring balance to your tone. If you're just getting started with it, use a lower strength and gradually build up to let your skin adjust comfortably.

Cleansing

Cleansing is the starting point of any skincare routine and plays a big part in helping your skin stay fresh and balanced. Before applying any other product, it's important to clean your face thoroughly to remove makeup, oil, dirt, and other buildup that can block the effect of anything applied afterward. Instead of bar soap, which can throw off your skin's natural balance—especially if it's not designed for the face—go for a product meant for facial use. Bar soaps not made for delicate skin can leave it dry or even allow yeast and bacteria to grow more easily. Some people think foam is a sign that something's working, but a strong lather can actually take away too much of your skin's natural oils. Dermatologist Erum Ilyas explained that the ingredients that cause foaming can make it harder for your skin's surface to stay in good shape. This was also backed by a study in 2012, which found that some cleansing agents disturb how skin cells are meant to stay organized.

Stick to lukewarm water when washing your face. Hot water won't "open" your pores, and cold water doesn't "close" them. The idea that pores work like doors isn't accurate. What hot water does do is cause irritation, especially if your skin is already sensitive. Micellar water is another good option, especially if you're traveling or don't have access to clean running water. It contains small cleansing molecules called micelles that attach to oil and dirt, lifting them from the skin. For those who don't wear makeup daily, micellar water can sometimes serve as a complete cleanser on its own and doesn't need to be rinsed off. Skip tools like sponges and loofahs, which can collect bacteria unless constantly disinfected. The cleanest tools you can use are your own hands—just make sure you wash them first. Also, don't forget areas like your neck and jawline, which are just as exposed to buildup and need attention, too. A light upward massage while cleansing can also help with circulation and give your face a break from the tension of the day.

When drying your face, pat gently using a clean, soft towel. Letting water drip dry might seem like a good idea, but once it evaporates, it can take moisture from your skin along with it, leaving you feeling drier than before. Try not to wash your face more than needed. If you already cleanse in the shower, adding another wash twice a day at the sink might be too much. For those with dry or sensitive skin, cutting back can make a difference. And when it comes to timing your nighttime wash, earlier might be better. There's research suggesting that syncing with your skin's natural rhythm can help keep it looking its best—so consider washing your face before the sun sets.

Lastly, make sure you're using the right amount of cleanser. Sometimes when a product doesn't seem to work, it's just that not enough is being used. It can be tempting to stretch out pricey products by using less than suggested, but this can affect the outcome. Always check the label for the recommended amount, since products are usually tested to work best within those guidelines.

Types of Cleanser for different skins

There are many options when it comes to facial cleansers—from smooth clay-based formulas to balms that gently break down even stubborn makeup. Understanding the different types can help you choose what suits your skin best.

Gel cleansers are water-based with a slippery, jelly-like feel. They provide a deep clean while remaining gentle enough not to strip your skin's natural oils. Many are made with ingredients like glycerin or hyaluronic acid to support hydration. To use one, wet your face and hands with lukewarm water, create a foamy lather, massage it into your skin in circles, then rinse and pat dry. Gel formulas are well-suited for oily or acne-prone skin, and they also work well as a follow-up cleanse after using a balm or oil.

Cream cleansers have a smooth, rich texture that produces a satisfying lather. Like gels, they are water-based but often include moisturizing oils such as shea butter or jojoba oil. These are best applied to damp skin and followed with a light massage and rinse. Their nourishing nature makes them ideal for dry or combination skin and those seeking a gentler wash than an oil-based product. Oil cleansers are entirely oil-based and come in both liquid and balm forms. Applied to dry skin, they lift away makeup, dirt, and excess oil. The oil binds to debris and is then washed away with water. There are two approaches: a basic oil cleanse using warm water and a soft cloth, or the popular double cleanse, which follows up with a gentle water-based wash. Those with dry or combination skin often find oil cleansers leave a comforting layer of moisture. For anyone worried about leftover residue, pairing with a gel or foaming cleanser helps remove any trace.

Foam cleansers feel light and airy. While older versions could be drying, newer ones are much gentler. Often, the foam comes from the pump, not harsh additives. Start by rinsing your face with warm water, then massage the foam in for up to a minute before rinsing. Always pat dry with a soft towel. Foam cleansers are a solid pick for those with oily or blemish-prone skin. Clay cleansers are built on ingredients like kaolin or bentonite, known for drawing out excess oil. These have a thick, muddy texture and work well to reduce shine and improve the look of pores. Use them once daily or a few times a week, depending on your skin type. Mix with water, apply in circles, then rinse thoroughly.

Powder cleansers come dry and are activated with water to form a paste. They often include exfoliating bits like rice powder or clay. How much water you add can change the texture—less makes it scrubby, more makes it soft. Massage it in and rinse it away with lukewarm water. This type works great for oily or travel-friendly routines since it contains no liquids. Micellar water was made popular in France and works like a magnet for makeup and dirt. The micelles within bind to debris and whisk it away—no rinsing required. Just soak a cotton pad and swipe across the face. It's suitable for all skin types and perfect for those who want a gentle cleanse without needing a sink. It also works well as a pre-cleanser before using a gel or foam.

Bar cleansers are solid soaps designed for the face. Unlike traditional body bars, these are often made with moisturizing and creamy ingredients. Rub between your hands to create a lather, apply to your face, and rinse well. Stick to bars made specifically for facial use to avoid drying effects.

Balm cleansers melt away makeup and impurities while giving your skin a soft, pampered feel. When mixed with water, they often turn milky and rinse clean. Use dry hands to apply the balm to dry skin, massage in circular strokes, add water to emulsify, then rinse. These are best for normal to dry skin due to their soothing oils like shea butter or grapeseed.

Cleansing wipes and pads are convenient for travel or end-of-day routines. Pre-soaked with cleansing solutions, they remove oil and makeup in seconds. While handy, they may not always be gentle, especially those with alcohol. Look for ones with calming ingredients like aloe or micellar water, and use them gently across your face. Always follow up with a full cleanse if using wipes alone. Each of these cleansers offers something different, and finding the right one comes down to your skin type, lifestyle and what your skin responds to best.

Best cleanser active ingredients for different skins

Salicylic acid

Reducing breakouts and clearing blocked pores.

Beta hydroxy acid works deep within the skin, reaching into the pores to clean out buildup and remove debris that often leads to pimples. It's a solid choice for those who struggle with acne or skin congestion. When added to a face wash, it helps calm areas of redness and swelling around blemishes while also helping prevent new ones from forming. If you're dealing with active spots, this ingredient can make a noticeable difference in how your skin looks and feels.

Hyaluronic acid

Hyaluronic acid works well for anyone looking to support their skin's moisture balance. Some face cleansers can strip away natural oils, leaving the skin feeling dry and tight. Hyaluronic acid, known as a humectant, helps by attracting water from the air and drawing it into the skin, keeping it soft and comfortable. It forms a lightweight layer that holds moisture in, making the skin feel smooth and fresh. Cleansers containing hyaluronic acid are especially good for dry or sensitive skin, offering lasting hydration without irritation.

Niacinamide

Niacinamide is a multi-tasking ingredient that works well for those with oily or uneven skin. It helps balance oil on the surface, which can reduce the look of enlarged pores and help calm breakouts. This ingredient also supports a brighter complexion by reducing the look of dark spots and uneven tone. In addition to these benefits, niacinamide helps keep the skin's outer layer strong and better protected from outside factors that may cause dryness or irritation.

Vitamin C

Vitamin C is known for helping brighten skin, even out tone, and fade marks like sunspots or areas of discoloration. It also supports collagen production, which helps keep your skin firm and smooth. This ingredient plays a key role in keeping your skin looking fresh and less affected by daily wear. However, because it's quite active, those with dry or reactive skin may want to use it just a few times a week instead of applying it every day.

Ceramides

Ceramides play a big part in keeping your skin firm and well-moisturized. They help maintain the outer layer, which acts like a shield—holding in moisture and blocking out unwanted irritants. This ingredient is suitable for all skin types and supports smooth, soft skin with a fresh appearance. It's especially helpful in preventing dryness and keeping your skin looking full and refreshed.

AHAs

Alpha hydroxy acids (AHAs), such as glycolic and lactic acid, offer a smooth way to remove buildup from the skin. If you're looking for a cleanser that gently clears away old skin cells while also keeping your skin feeling fresh, AHAs can help. They work well to lift away impurities without being too rough, making them a good match for sensitive skin types.

Colloidal oatmeal

Colloidal oatmeal, drawn from finely ground oats, is a gentle and comforting ingredient often found in facial cleansers. Known for its soothing nature, it helps calm skin that's feeling irritated or dry. Rich in naturally calming compounds, it helps ease discomfort and supports the skin's ability to stay balanced. Alongside its soothing effects, it also helps keep moisture in and supports a healthy surface by maintaining the skin's natural pH.

Squalane

Squalane, a lighter and more stable form of squalene, is a skin-friendly oil that helps lock in moisture. It closely resembles the natural oils found in the skin, making it well-tolerated and effective at maintaining hydration without feeling heavy. Along with keeping the skin soft and smooth, it also helps protect against everyday exposure that can wear the skin down. It works well across all skin types, including oily, dry, or sensitive.

Micellar water

Micellar water is a gentle and effective option for those with sensitive, dry, or acne-prone skin. It's especially useful for clearing away makeup at the end of the day. When a specific level of surfactant is mixed with water, it forms tiny cleansing bubbles called micelles. These micelles attract and lift away oil, makeup, and impurities while also keeping the skin feeling soft and hydrated.

Benzoyl Peroxide

Benzoyl peroxide is widely used to manage acne because of how well it targets the source of breakouts. It works by clearing away the bacteria responsible for acne, known as Cutibacterium acnes, while also helping to unclog pores by removing extra oil and dead skin buildup. This combination reduces both the presence of bacteria and excess sebum, making it especially helpful for people with oily skin who experience frequent breakouts.

Peptides

Peptides are short chains formed from amino acids, which are the basic components of proteins. Cleansers that contain peptides can be used by anyone, but they're especially useful for skin that feels dry, shows early signs of aging, or tends to react easily. These ingredients are favored because they absorb well and support the skin in several ways, such as helping it hold on to moisture and reducing the look of fine lines.

Steps for Cleansing

Cleansing your face is a key step in any skincare routine. While it might seem straightforward, how you wash your face actually matters. Taking the time to do it properly can help your skin look clear and feel refreshed, while skipping steps or rushing through it may lead to breakouts or buildup over time.

Most people believe cleansing is only necessary when wearing makeup or when the skin looks dirty, but it's best to wash your face twice daily. That said, how well you clean your skin often matters more than how often. Regardless of whether your skin is dry, oily, or in between, washing it at night is especially important. It helps remove leftover makeup, dirt, and oils, giving your skin a clean surface to absorb your evening products and allowing it to rest and recover overnight.

If you're ready to give your face the proper care it needs, following the right steps during cleansing can make all the difference.

Step 1: Firstly, thoroughly remove all of your makeup or sunscreen.

During the day, your skin may have been covered with layers of makeup or, at the very least, sunscreen. Before washing your face—especially at night—it's important to take off these products first. Starting with a gentle makeup remover helps clear the surface, allowing your cleanser to work more effectively.

At night, your skin works to push out waste through the pores. If they're blocked, the buildup stays trapped, leading to a congested look and feel. This applies to every skin type, even if your skin tends to be thicker or tougher on the surface. A clean start is the best way to support your skin's natural recovery while you sleep.

Step 2: Apply an oil-based cleanser or any cleanser of your choice.

Using a regular face wash alone may not be enough since your skin collects different kinds of buildup throughout the day. To fully remove layers of oil and grime, an oil-based cleanser can be helpful. These cleansers are made to break down excess sebum without stripping away the skin's natural moisture, leaving your face clean but still comfortable.

Step 3: Use a water-based cleaner.

Your face-cleansing process should also include a water-based cleanser. This type of product helps clear away anything that might remain on your skin after the first step, such as sweat or other debris that dissolves in water. It's an important part of making sure your skin is fully clean and ready for the next steps in your routine.

Step 4: Exfoliate (optional).

If cleansing alone doesn't feel like it's doing enough, you can include exfoliation in your routine. This step is completely optional, but it can help lift away buildup on the skin's surface.

Take it easy when exfoliating: Rubbing too hard can wear down your skin's natural defenses. A light touch with your fingertips for a minute or two is all you need. To exfoliate, choose products that list lactic acid, salicylic acid, glycolic acid, or fruit enzymes. Letting them sit on your skin for around 60 to 90 seconds helps clean out pores and remove dead cells, leaving your face feeling fresh and smooth.

Step 5: Put toner or essence.

After cleansing, the next step is applying toner. Toners help provide light hydration and can refresh the skin, making it ready to take in the next steps in your routine. They can also support skin balance and include ingredients that serve different needs. Although toners were once used mainly to help your skin maintain a healthy pH level, many now also contain ingredients that care for specific concerns.

- Some helpful ingredients to look for include:
- Rosewater, known for its skin-softening qualities.
- Chamomile, often used to calm stressed skin.

- Witch hazel or salicylic acid, which are useful if you deal with breakouts.

To apply, pour a small amount onto a cotton pad and gently sweep it over areas such as the forehead, nose, and chin.

Step 6: Moisturize and/or apply serum.

Once you've washed your face, it's important to restore moisture to keep your skin soft and balanced. A good way to do this is by using a moisturizer that fits your skin's hydration needs. Try to choose one that provides enough moisture without feeling thick or greasy. If the product is too rich, it may block your pores and lead to breakouts. The goal is to find something that keeps your skin feeling smooth and fresh without weighing it down.

Step 7: Complete with eye cream and lip balm.

Complete your cleansing routine by applying an eye cream. This step helps care for the delicate skin around your eyes, which can easily show signs of tiredness. Eye creams are helpful for reducing the look of puffiness and dark areas. While you're caring for your face, remember to treat your lips as well. Dry, cracked lips can draw attention away from the rest of your face. A good lip balm can keep them soft, smooth, and looking healthy.

Exfoliating, Why and How to Do It Safely

Exfoliation involves removing dead skin cells from the outer layer of the skin. While some people find that it improves how their skin looks, it's not the best option for everyone. When done the wrong way, it can lead to irritation, redness, or even more breakouts. If you choose to exfoliate, it's important to do it with care to avoid harming your skin. Not all exfoliating techniques work well for every skin type, so it's a good idea to consider what suits your skin before picking a method.

At-home exfoliation can be done in two main ways: mechanical or chemical, and the right choice depends on your skin's needs. Mechanical exfoliation involves using tools like brushes, sponges or scrubs to physically remove dead skin. Chemical exfoliation uses ingredients such as alpha hydroxy acids (AHAs) or beta hydroxy acids (BHAs) to gently lift away dead cells.

Exfoliating helps for several reasons.

It helps your skin look brighter. Normally, your skin renews itself around every four weeks. As this process slows down with age, dead skin tends to build up, leaving your face looking rough and dry. Regular exfoliation clears away these dull layers, allowing fresher skin to come through and bringing back a natural glow.

It helps keep your pores clear. Exfoliating removes buildup that your daily face wash might miss. When pores are kept clean, they appear smaller, and your chances of dealing with breakouts are lower.

It helps your skincare work better. Dead skin and clogged pores can make it harder for your products to be absorbed properly. Once that layer is removed, your skin can take in moisture and other care products more effectively.

It makes your skin feel smoother and can reduce uneven tone. Dry patches and buildup can cause roughness or dark areas. Exfoliating helps smooth out the surface and create a more even look.

It helps makeup go on more evenly. When your skin is clean and smooth, your makeup sits better. Foundation is less likely to clump or settle into dry spots, giving a smoother finish.

Exfoliating by Skin Type

When exfoliating by hand, it's important to treat your skin with care. Apply the scrub gently using your fingertips in small, circular motions. You can also use a soft brush or tool of your choice, keeping the strokes short and light. Limit this step to around thirty seconds, then rinse your face with lukewarm water—never hot, as that may cause irritation. If your skin is cut, irritated, or sunburned, skip exfoliating until it heals. After you're done, apply a moisturizer that contains sun protection to keep your skin hydrated and shielded.

Dry skin: Exfoliation can help manage dry, flaky skin, but it's important to choose the right approach. Using scrubs or rough tools on dry skin may do more harm than good, as they can lead to irritation or tiny surface injuries. A gentler option is alpha hydroxy acids (AHAs), such as glycolic acid, which help lift away dead skin and support skin renewal. After using products with glycolic acid, it's important to apply both sunscreen and moisturizer, as the skin may be more likely to react to sunlight.

Sensitive skin: Avoid using scrubs or rough tools on your skin, as these can lead to irritation and increase redness. Instead, choose a mild chemical exfoliant paired with a soft cloth to gently clean the surface. For acne-related concerns, a salicylic acid peel provided by your dermatologist may help support clearer skin without causing further discomfort.

Oily skin: Mechanical exfoliation and gentle brushing can be helpful for skin that tends to feel greasy or appear thick. This type of skin often has a buildup on the surface, which physical exfoliation can help remove. For best results, apply your scrub or exfoliating product using small, circular strokes, taking your time to work it across your skin evenly.

Normal skin: If your skin isn't dealing with any major concerns, you have the flexibility to try different exfoliation methods. Both physical and chemical options can work well. It may take a bit of trial and error to figure out which one feels and performs best on your skin.

Combination skin: For combination skin, you might find that using both physical and chemical exfoliation works well, depending on the areas you're targeting. However, avoid applying both methods on the same day, as this can lead to irritation. If your skin feels dry afterward, follow up with a moisturizer right away to keep it comfortable and balanced.

Exfoliation by Body Part

When exfoliating sensitive areas like the face, it's important to go gently. Overdoing it can lead to dryness, redness, or irritation. Treat these spots with care to keep your skin calm and balanced.

Face: The type of exfoliant you use on your face should match your skin's needs. For a scrub, gently apply it with your fingertips and move in small circles. Rinse with lukewarm water when done. If you're using a liquid exfoliant, it's best to apply it with a cotton pad or soft cloth. To know what's best for your skin, consider speaking with a skincare professional.

Arms and Legs: To exfoliate your arms and legs, using a glove, sponge, or brush is one of the easiest approaches. This helps remove buildup on the skin and can also encourage better blood flow. Look for a body scrub either in a nearby store or through an online shop, and apply it during your shower. You can also consider using a dry brush before bathing for similar results.

Feet and Hands: You can find both scrubs and peels designed to smooth the skin on your hands and feet. Another useful option for your feet is a pumice stone, which can help gently remove rough or dry areas during your regular care routine.

Pubic area: Use a soft towel or a body brush to gently clean around the bikini line and nearby areas. Make sure to do this while taking a warm shower, which helps soften the skin. Apply the scrub with care, using light strokes, and rinse off completely when finished.

Avoiding Skin Injury During Exfoliating

Check the products you're already using on your skin. Some treatments—both prescription and store-bought, like retinoid creams or lotions with benzoyl peroxide—can make your skin more prone to dryness or irritation. Adding exfoliation while using these may make dryness worse or lead to breakouts.

Choose a method of exfoliation that matches your skin's needs. If your skin is dry, sensitive, or prone to acne, go for a soft cloth paired with a mild chemical exfoliant. Scrubs may feel too harsh. If your skin is thicker or more oily, you might do better with a stronger chemical formula or a physical exfoliant. Those with deeper skin tones or skin that marks easily after irritation should avoid anything too aggressive, as it could cause dark spots to form.

Use a gentle touch. Whether you're applying a scrub or a chemical formula, rub lightly in small circles for about half a minute, then rinse with warm—not hot—water. If you're using a sponge or brush, keep the strokes short and soft. Avoid exfoliating over sunburn, cuts, or other open areas.

Moisturize afterward. Since exfoliating can remove some of the skin's moisture, following up with a good moisturizer helps keep your skin feeling smooth and hydrated.

Figure out how often your skin needs exfoliation. The right schedule depends on your skin type and what kind of exfoliant you're using. Stronger treatments should be spaced out more, while milder ones can be done more often. Doing it too frequently may cause redness or sensitivity.

Moisturizing by Skin Type

Moisturizers are key in supporting healthy skin by helping it stay hydrated and reinforcing its natural barrier. Whether your skin is dry, oily, or somewhere in between, staying properly moisturized can help prevent rough texture, flaking, and early signs of aging. One important ingredient to look for is hyaluronic acid, which holds a high amount of water and helps the skin stay soft and smooth. Products made with natural and plant-based ingredients are often gentler and less likely to cause reactions. Using the right moisturizer regularly can keep your skin balanced and leave it looking fresh and well-cared for. When choosing a moisturizer, it's important to consider what your skin truly needs. Each skin type benefits from different textures and ingredients, so understanding your skin's condition will help you pick what works best.

Dry Skin: To care for dry skin effectively, it's important to use a moisturizer that matches your skin's specific needs. Dry skin often requires more support to stay smooth and hydrated, so choosing the right product can make a big difference. Look for moisturizers that include ingredients like hyaluronic acid and glycerin, as they help draw moisture into the skin and keep it from escaping. Cream-based moisturizers tend to work better for dry skin, as they offer lasting hydration and create a layer that helps hold moisture in. Products labeled with terms like "moisturizing," "nourishing," or "hydrating" are often made to support dry skin and can improve both comfort and appearance.

Oily Skin: For oily skin, the focus should be on finding a moisturizer that hydrates without making your skin greasy. Look for oil-free options that won't block pores and that feel light when applied. Hyaluronic acid can help add moisture without making the skin feel heavy, while niacinamide supports better balance by helping manage oil levels. Gel or water-based products are great choices because they absorb quickly and don't leave a shiny finish. Try to stay away from thick creams or anything containing mineral oils, as these can add to the oiliness and may lead to clogged pores.

Combination Skin: Choosing a suitable moisturizer for combination skin means finding one that provides enough hydration to dry areas without making oily zones feel greasy. It's important to go with products that can support both needs without clogging pores or increasing shine.

Pick lightweight options like oil-free or gel-textured moisturizers. These can refresh oily spots, especially the T-zone, without adding extra oil.

Focus on hydrating ingredients like hyaluronic acid or glycerin. These help soften dry patches while keeping the skin feeling smooth.

A daily moisturizer with at least SPF 30 can protect against sun damage without making your skin appear shiny or heavy.

Sensitive Skin: Choosing the right moisturizer for sensitive skin means focusing on formulas that are gentle and free from common triggers. Look for products labeled as hypoallergenic, fragrance-free, and non-comedogenic to help avoid unwanted reactions. Moisturizers containing aloe vera, ceramides, colloidal oatmeal, or hyaluronic acid can help calm and support the skin while keeping it soft and comfortable. These ingredients are known to support hydration and help reduce dryness without irritating the skin.

Stay away from harsh ingredients like alcohol, dyes, artificial scents, and harsh preservatives. These can lead to discomfort, redness, or flaking. It's a good idea to do a patch test before using any new product—try it on a small area first to make sure your skin responds well. When caring for sensitive skin, keeping your routine simple is often best. Stick to moisturizers that contain gentle, hydrating ingredients like glycerin and hyaluronic acid. Avoid anything with sulfates, parabens, or synthetic perfumes that might disturb your skin's balance.

Key ingredients to search for in moisturizers

To find the right moisturizer for your skin, focus on those that contain ingredients known for supporting hydration and skin balance.

• Hyaluronic acid draws moisture into the skin and helps keep it fresh without feeling heavy or greasy.

• Glycerin works by locking in water, helping your skin stay soft and preventing dryness.

• Ceramides are lipids that support your skin's outer layer, helping it stay strong, retain moisture, and resist daily stress.

When picking a moisturizer, consider options that are not tested on animals and include plant-based extracts, gentle oils, and natural ingredients. These additions may offer added comfort for the skin and can address different skin concerns without being harsh.

Sunscreen

Sunscreen plays a key role in keeping your skin protected from harmful rays from the sun. It helps guard against sunburn, signs of aging, and skin cancer. Using sunscreen regularly is one of the easiest ways to support your skin's condition and appearance through the years. When applied as part of your routine, it helps reduce the chances of damage caused by long-term sun exposure. To pick the right sunscreen, choose one with at least SPF 30 for daily use. If you plan to be outside for long periods, go for SPF 60 or higher. Most people don't apply enough sunscreen, so using a higher SPF helps cover that gap. For full coverage of areas like the face, neck, arms, and legs, you'll need about one ounce of sunscreen. That's roughly the amount that would fill your entire palm. For just your face and neck, around half a teaspoon should be enough.

Sunscreen protects your skin by forming a barrier against the sun's rays. It's designed to block both UVA and UVB rays, which can harm skin cells and break down proteins like collagen and elastin—this leads to wrinkles and other visible changes over time. Some sunscreens work by absorbing into the top layers of skin and trapping UV rays before they do damage. These often include ingredients such as homosalate. Others sit on top of the skin and reflect sunlight; these are made with minerals like zinc oxide or titanium dioxide. Some products combine both methods for extra protection.

Benefits of Sunscreen

Sunscreen plays a key role in shielding your skin from the sun's harmful rays. As the ozone layer becomes thinner, the chances of getting sunburn and other damage from UV exposure increase. A sunscreen with a high SPF helps block these rays, especially when used on both the face and body. Look for one that protects against both UVA and UVB rays, since both types contribute to long-term skin problems and raise the risk of skin cancer. Wearing sunscreen every day can also support your skin's long-term well-being. A simple habit like applying it regularly can help prevent skin-related conditions. Adding sunscreen to your daily care routine is a smart move that goes a long way in protecting your skin's surface. Exposure to sunlight can cause the skin to lose its smooth appearance. UV rays break down collagen, leading to wrinkles and sagging. Over time, repeated exposure without protection can lead to early signs of aging. Those who apply sunscreen regularly are less likely to deal with fine lines and sagging in the long run.

Even skin tone is another benefit of consistent sunscreen use. Uneven color, including dark spots, can make the skin appear older. Applying sunscreen helps maintain an even tone and leaves the skin looking fresh. This small step can be part of your morning routine. If you use other skincare products, apply sunscreen last, just before any makeup. It helps you keep a smooth and fresh appearance with minimal effort. Sunscreen also builds a layer of protection that defends against sun-related changes in the skin. With continued use, it can reduce the chance of changes like creases, patches, and other visible concerns. This protection helps your skin stay clearer for longer.

Burns caused by too much sun can lead to rough texture and a dull look. Sunscreen helps protect your skin by lowering the risk of damage from the sun's rays, which helps preserve its smooth feel. It also helps reduce the chance of dark patches developing in areas exposed to sunlight. In some cases, sun exposure leads to small dark spots known as sunspots. Daily sunscreen application can help reduce the chance of these appearing by shielding the skin from the sun's impact. It also helps in managing melasma, a condition that causes patches of dark skin, usually on the face. Applying sunscreen each day may help stop the condition from getting worse. Many sunscreen formulas contain ingredients that keep the skin feeling soft and hydrated. Since dry skin can be more easily affected by sun exposure, keeping your skin moisturized adds another layer of protection against damage.

Types of Sun Screens and Their Protective Level

There are two main types of sunscreen: mineral (also known as physical) and chemical. Mineral sunscreen stays on the surface of the skin and acts as a shield, reflecting sunlight in a way similar to how tiny mirrors bounce light away. These products are known to help block both UVA and UVB rays. They usually contain titanium dioxide, zinc oxide, or a blend of both. Since these formulas work right where they are applied, they begin to protect immediately. However, they may need to be reapplied often and can sometimes leave a slight white layer on the skin.

On the other hand, chemical sunscreens work below the skin's top layer. They absorb the sun's rays and convert them into heat before releasing them. Ingredients like avobenzone, octisalate, oxybenzone, homosalate, and others are used in these products. Since chemical sunscreens need to sink in to be effective, they should be applied about 20 minutes before heading outside. These options are also known to resist water better and absorb quickly without leaving residue. Choosing the right sunscreen depends on your skin's needs:

For oily skin: Lighter, water-based chemical sunscreens usually feel less greasy and are a better match than oil-based options.

For dry skin: Look for sunscreens that include moisturizing elements like glycerin, ceramides, or hyaluronic acid. Some products combine sun protection and hydration in one.

For skin prone to breakouts: Mineral sunscreens are often a good pick. Titanium dioxide and zinc oxide are less likely to block pores, and zinc may help calm redness.

For sensitive skin: Mineral sunscreens are more suitable here too, as chemical filters can warm the skin and cause discomfort.

For combination skin: A gel-based sunscreen can help manage oily spots without drying out the rest of the face.

For balanced skin: Those with no dryness or extra oiliness can choose either type, depending on personal preference.

In terms of strength, protection levels can be described as:

Low: under SPF 15

Medium: SPF 15 to 29

High: SPF 30 to 49

Very high: SPF 50 and above

This labeling is more common in regions outside the U.S., though SPF numbers are still displayed. Sunscreen also comes in several forms. In addition to lotions, you can choose:

- Creams
- Gels
- Sticks
- Sprays

Each one offers a different feel and application style, allowing you to find something that fits comfortably into your routine.

Anti-Aging Routine

When building an anti-aging skincare routine, it's important to focus on ingredients that have a solid track record of supporting skin health over time. A simple routine doesn't need to be complicated, but it should include products that help care for your skin gently while also addressing common signs of aging.

Starting with a mild cleanser is key. Washing your face at least once daily is non-negotiable, especially at night. If you can manage to cleanse both morning and evening, that's even better, but once a day is the bare minimum to remove buildup and keep your skin fresh.

One ingredient that has received a lot of attention for its role in both skin health and immune support is vitamin C. In skincare, vitamin C can help even out skin tone and bring back a brighter look to tired skin. It's a common ingredient in many serums designed to fight signs of age, and for good reason—it supports skin's natural renewal process while helping to reduce the look of discoloration.

Retinol is another well-known part of many anti-aging routines. Often referred to as vitamin A or in some cases by its medical name, retinoid, this ingredient has long been favored for its ability to improve skin texture and reduce the appearance of fine lines. Though strong, it can be very effective when introduced gradually and paired with other skin-soothing products.

Keeping skin well hydrated is also an important part of slowing visible aging. As the skin grows older, it tends to produce less oil, which often results in dryness. Adding a face lotion or cream that fits your skin type can help bring back softness and smoothness. In many cases, a good moisturizer also adds a temporary plumpness to the skin, helping it appear smoother and reducing the look of lines.

Of all the products in your routine, sunscreen might be the most important. According to many skin experts, using sunscreen daily—not just in warm months or on sunny days—is one of the best ways to help your skin stay youthful. Sun damage is a major cause of early aging, so applying broad-spectrum sunscreen every morning is a small step that can make a big difference over time.

Chapter Four

Enhancing Your Routine

Most people skip serums in their skincare routine, often because they assume these products are either just another moisturizer or not worth the effort. In truth, that's far from accurate. A well-chosen serum can make a noticeable difference and support the overall effectiveness of your routine. A facial serum is a lightweight product that contains a higher level of active ingredients than your standard face cream. These ingredients—such as hyaluronic acid, vitamin C, niacinamide, glycolic acid, and salicylic acid—are included for their ability to target specific skin concerns in a concentrated way. There are different types of serums, each formulated to focus on a particular issue. Some are made to deeply hydrate the skin and improve its softness, which makes them a good fit for those with dryness. Others work well in managing uneven tone or texture, helping to brighten dull areas and soften rough patches. Some serums are better suited for managing breakouts or calming red, irritated spots. Others can help improve the look of fine lines, soften wrinkles, and support smoother texture with regular use.

What sets serums apart from other skincare products is their ability to go deeper into the skin's surface due to their lightweight and fast-absorbing nature. Because of this, they're often used to deliver targeted care for things like dehydration, dark marks, uneven tone, or roughness. Using a serum can improve the results of the rest of your skincare steps. When applied to freshly washed skin, just a few drops are usually enough. Let it absorb for a moment, then follow up with a moisturizer. If you're using a product during the day, don't forget to finish with sun protection to help maintain your skin's condition and prevent further concerns from developing. Including a serum in your daily care can help give your skin the extra support it needs, whether you're aiming for better hydration, smoother texture, or a more even appearance. The key is choosing one that matches what your skin needs at the time and giving it a chance to work consistently.

Facial Oils

Face oils are nourishing blends made from plant-based sources that provide the skin with lasting moisture and care. Packed with antioxidants, essential fats, and vitamins, they help support a well-balanced skin barrier and may soften signs of aging over time. Depending on the specific oil, they can suit different skin needs—including sensitive types—by improving softness, helping reduce the appearance of fine lines, and giving the skin a natural glow. These oils can work in two key ways: by softening the surface and by forming a layer that holds in moisture. Each oil offers its own set of nutrients that help keep the skin looking smooth and refreshed by supporting the outer protective layer of the skin, also known as the stratum corneum. For example, coconut oil is known for its deep moisture, jojoba oil for its softening properties, and rosehip oil for its ability to support skin clarity and tone with its natural antioxidants.

Face Oil Based On Skin Types

Normal Skin

Argan Oil: Argan oil is often called "liquid gold" because of the wide range of benefits it offers the skin. This rich and calming oil is packed with vitamin E, a nutrient known for its protective properties. It helps reduce the appearance of dark spots, fine lines, and other skin concerns by supporting overall skin balance and comfort.

Aside from its use in skincare, argan oil is also a helpful solution for hair. If you're dealing with frizz or split ends, it can be used as a conditioning treatment. It's known to smooth the strands and leave hair looking soft and glossy. Whether applied to the skin or hair, a few drops can go a long way in maintaining a healthy and refreshed look.

Squalene Oil: Squalene is a natural oil found in olives, rice bran, and even produced by your own skin. On its own, though, it breaks down quickly when exposed to air and can sometimes block pores. Squalane, a more stable version of squalene, is often used in skincare instead. It shares a similar structure with the oils your skin produces, which means it is absorbed easily without leaving a heavy residue.

Because of how well it works with the skin, squalane helps address dryness and supports a smoother texture. It's also known to support collagen activity, helping skin feel firmer and look more refreshed. Whether your skin is dry, tired, or in need of balance, a few drops can bring back softness and a more even appearance.

Retinol Oil: Retinol oils help keep your skin hydrated, even out your tone, and clear up occasional breakouts without causing irritation. They offer a gentle way to smooth the surface of your skin while supporting a fresh, clean look. Even when your skin isn't at its best, these oils can support a steady routine that brings things back into balance without being too harsh or drying.

Dry Skin

Marula Oil: Marula oil contains omega-rich fats that help keep dry skin soft and smooth. It delivers lasting moisture and may help calm redness or irritation. One of its best features is how light it feels—absorbing quickly without leaving a greasy layer behind.

Almond oil: Almond oil has long been used to care for dry skin conditions such as eczema, psoriasis, and dermatitis. Packed with vitamin A, it may also support the renewal of skin, helping to soften fine lines over time. Its gentle nature makes it a popular choice for improving skin texture, though anyone with a nut allergy should avoid applying it to prevent unwanted reactions.

Avocado oil: Avocado facial oil supplies the skin with nutrients like potassium, vitamin E, and lecithin, which help keep dryness under control. These elements absorb well into the outer layer of the skin, supporting the renewal of fresh skin cells and helping the surface stay soft and smooth.

Oily Skin

Peppermint Oil: Peppermint is a reliable ingredient found in many face oils, known for helping to balance oil levels and keeping pores from getting blocked. Adding this to your skincare routine can help reduce breakouts and keep your skin clearer. It's also known for its cooling and soothing feel, making it useful for calming redness or easing the sting of mild burns.

Grape Seed Oil: Grapeseed oil is a plant-based ingredient that helps manage excess shine by lifting away extra oil from your skin. It can also make your pores look tighter, giving your face a smoother, less glossy finish.

Tea Tree Oil: Tea tree oil is a helpful option for those with oily skin, thanks to its natural ability to fight off bacteria and fungus. It can reach below the skin's surface, helping to clear blocked pores and balance oil production, which may leave your skin feeling cleaner and more refreshed.

Acne-Prone Skin

Pomegranate Oil: Pomegranate oil works to target the bacteria that build up in your pores and lead to breakouts and irritation. It's a great match for oily skin since it's light in texture and won't leave behind a greasy look or feel.

Rosehip Oil: Rosehip oil contains a rich blend of skin-friendly vitamins and essential fatty acids, making it a helpful choice for calming irritated skin and managing breakouts. It also has phenols, which are known for their antibacterial and antifungal properties, all without clogging the pores. This oil is often used to improve the appearance of old acne marks and reduce overall redness. Interestingly, a 2015 study found rosehip oil to be effective in helping scars heal after surgery.

Coconut Oil: Coconut oil offers natural properties that help fight off bacteria and reduce the appearance of inflamed breakouts. It's also useful as a gentle cleansing option for the face, helping to lift away dirt while loosening debris from the pores. By using it this way, your skin can feel cleaner and look more refreshed over time.

Combination Skin

Jojoba Oil: Jojoba oil works well to break down and dissolve excess sebum, which helps control oily patches on the face. At the same time, it provides hydration to drier spots without clogging pores. Its light texture allows it to sit comfortably on the skin, making it a good match for those dealing with both dry and oily areas. This balance makes it especially helpful for people who have combination skin.

Marula Oil: Marula oil offers a natural way to support your skin's defense against daily exposure to dirt, smoke, and other outside stressors. Its quick-absorbing texture allows it to work well as a hydrating option without leaving a greasy finish. Regular use can help balance the skin's natural oil levels while keeping it soft and smooth.

Flaxseed Oil: Flaxseed oil, rich in healthy fats, is a gentle option for calming breakouts and easing dryness. It supports the skin's ability to hold onto moisture, helping it stay soft and well-hydrated. Over time, it may also help smooth out lines, fade dark areas, and reduce puffiness. If you're looking for a simple makeup remover that won't cause irritation, flaxseed oil can be a great natural choice.

Sensitive Skin

Aloe Vera Oil: Aloe vera works well for people with sensitive skin because it's packed with calming agents, nourishing fats, and protective nutrients. It helps soothe irritation, defend the skin against unwanted bacteria, and support recovery when the skin feels stressed or damaged. Since it also has a natural tightening effect, it's a great option for those with delicate skin that's prone to breakouts.

Moringa Oil: Moringa oil, much like aloe vera, offers calming and nourishing effects that can help care for delicate skin. It's also a good choice when you need moisture without using something too heavy. Because of its light texture, it can be applied before makeup to keep dry or reactive skin feeling soft and smooth throughout the day.

Castor Oil: Castor oil can help reduce puffiness and swelling on the face. It's especially useful for calming irritated skin and easing the appearance of under-eye bags, giving your face a smoother, more refreshed look. Still, knowing which oil suits your skin is only part of the process. To truly benefit from it, you also need to use it the right way. Applying it correctly makes a big difference in how your skin responds and how well the oil works for you.

Tips to Get the Most from Face Oils

You can blend face oil with your moisturizer to add extra comfort to your skincare routine. If you're wondering about the right time to apply it, use face oil after any water-based products. Applying it after moisturizer helps seal in moisture and makes sure your skin absorbs the benefits of the oil more effectively. When applying, don't rub it into your skin. Instead, gently press it in with your fingertips—this prevents stress on your pores and allows the oil to sink in more easily.

You can also create your own blend by mixing different facial oils together. For instance, combining tea tree oil with lavender oil brings two distinct effects—tea tree helps manage acne, while lavender calms the skin. Even though some oils come in small bottles and may seem pricey, you only need a small amount—usually between three and six drops per use. If your skin feels drier than usual, adding an extra drop or two won't hurt.

Facial oils can do more than just moisturize your face. You can skip your regular eye cream and use a drop of oil instead. Since many face oils are plant-based and gentle, they're safe to use around sensitive areas like under the eyes. They also work well to hydrate dry lips—just pat a bit of oil over them to keep them soft and smooth. And if you want to give your brows and lashes some love, try adding a few drops there too. Argan oil, in particular, is known for its hair-conditioning qualities and may help them grow fuller with regular use.

Correct Application of Facial Oil and Benefits

To get the best results from your skincare products, the way you apply them matters just as much as the products themselves. Start by placing a few drops of oil into the palm of your hand—just a small amount is enough. Rub your hands together gently to warm the oil slightly, which helps it spread more easily. Then, press your palms lightly onto your face and neck, allowing the oil to settle into the skin without rubbing or dragging.

Using face oils regularly brings several benefits. They provide deep moisture, helping your skin stay soft and smooth throughout the day. These oils also feed the skin with nutrients it needs to stay healthy. Over time, they can support better skin texture, making it feel firmer and more flexible. If your skin is often irritated, many oils can help calm redness and discomfort. They also help manage your skin's natural oil, preventing it from becoming too greasy or too dry. And lastly, they give your face a soft, natural glow that makes your skin look more refreshed and alive.

Face Mask: Indulgence or Necessity?

A face mask is a thick cream or paste applied to the skin to help cleanse and smooth it. These masks often include vitamins, minerals, and natural ingredients like cactus or cucumber extracts that are known to be skin-friendly. Another form, the sheet mask, uses a thin layer of paper or fabric to deliver these ingredients directly to the face.

Adding a mask to your routine can bring noticeable benefits. It's not just a relaxing step—it can also target specific skin troubles. Whether you're dealing with dryness, breakouts, uneven skin tone, or lines, there's a mask that can help. With regular use, the right product can support cleaner, softer, and more balanced skin.

Types of Face Masks

Cream face masks have a texture that resembles thick moisturizer and are perfect for refreshing dry, tired, or mature skin. They help deliver extra moisture and nutrients, leaving the skin feeling soft and looking full. These masks are best applied to clean skin and used as a single treatment rather than part of a daily routine.

Gel masks feel smooth and light, similar to jam or jelly, making them a good choice for normal to oily skin. Some contain ingredients like raspberry or blackberry extracts that help control shine and tighten the look of pores. Others use natural hydrators like honey or stonecrop to comfort skin that feels dry or rough. If your skin feels hot or looks red, a gel mask can help bring it back to balance with its calming ingredients.

Clay masks are especially helpful for oily or acne-prone skin. The natural clay helps absorb excess oil, gently remove buildup, and calm irritated spots. Some clay masks, such as those made with charcoal, illite clay, and black seed oil, can help reduce the look of large pores and blemishes while leaving the skin feeling clean but not dry. They can also be applied to targeted areas instead of the whole face.

Exfoliating masks are designed to clear away dull surface cells and refresh your skin's appearance. These masks often come in the form of peels that include acids like AHAs or BHAs, which gently loosen and remove dead skin without harsh scrubbing.

Warming masks provide a tingling, warm feeling due to ingredients like cinnamon or paprika. This warmth comes from increased blood flow, which can give the skin a fresh look afterward. However, these are best avoided if your skin is easily irritated. A cream or gel formula would be a better fit for more delicate skin.

Sheet masks are simple and easy to use. They're made from soft fabrics soaked in liquid formulas packed with nutrients. Many include hydrating ingredients like hyaluronic acid along with plant-based extracts and vitamins. Each one targets a particular skin concern, and the materials used—like cotton, microfiber, or Tencel—help the mask sit comfortably on your face while delivering all the goodness it holds.

Face Mask Benefits and How to Use its

A face mask, much like a moisturizer or serum, is used to deliver skin-supporting ingredients in a more focused way. What sets it apart is how it forms a layer over your skin, locking in all the active ingredients and giving them time to work more deeply. While serums and creams are usually part of a daily routine, face masks are meant for occasional use when your skin could use some extra care. Depending on what your skin needs at the time, a mask can help by bringing back lost moisture, improving the way your skin feels, or making pores look smaller. It can also help clear out buildup, absorb oil, soften the look of lines, and improve firmness. For those dealing with uneven spots or dullness, a good mask can support a brighter and more even look, helping you feel refreshed and more comfortable in your skin.

Using the right mask for your skin is just the beginning—knowing how often to use it makes a big difference too. A good approach is to apply a face mask once or twice each week. Begin by cleansing and toning your skin first. These steps help remove dirt and excess oil, refresh your skin with a layer of hydration, and get it ready to absorb the goodness of your chosen mask. When you're ready to apply, spread the mask across your face in a smooth, even layer. It might seem like more product would work better, but a small amount—about the size of a cherry—is usually enough to cover your face. Don't forget to bring the product down to your neck and upper chest, areas that often get missed but are quick to show signs of dryness or aging.

Most masks are designed to stay on for around five to ten minutes, though it depends on the formula. Some are quick to work and should be rinsed off shortly after application, while others can stay on overnight for a more nourishing effect. Always check the product instructions to be sure you're using it as intended. When it's time to remove the mask, be gentle. Avoid harsh scrubbing or hot water, which can undo the benefits. Use lukewarm water and either rinse with your hands or gently wipe it away using a soft, clean cloth that won't cause friction or discomfort. Keeping your routine calm and simple helps your skin stay at its best.

Eye Creams: Targeting the Delicate Eye Area

Eye creams are moisturizers made specifically for the fragile skin around the eyes. Including one in your daily routine can help keep this area soft and prevent it from drying out. These creams support the skin's natural barrier and help the under-eye area appear smoother and firmer over time. When used regularly, they may reduce signs of tiredness and aging, like puffiness, fine lines, or shadows, while giving this delicate skin the care it needs.

Because the skin under the eyes is different from the rest of the face, it requires a more tailored approach. It tends to lose moisture quickly and is more prone to damage from sunlight and pollution. Repeated facial expressions like blinking or squinting also contribute to the formation of lines and creases. Unlike the rest of the face, the area under the eyes has fewer oil glands, so it needs extra help staying moisturized.

Eye creams are made with these factors in mind. They are often richer than regular face creams and contain more softening ingredients. Some are formulated with ingredients to reduce puffiness, such as caffeine, while others focus on softening the look of wrinkles using peptides. By choosing a cream made just for this part of the face and using it daily, you can better protect and care for the skin around your eyes.

Benefit of Eye Creams and How to Apply them

Eye creams can play an important role in refreshing the skin around your eyes, especially if puffiness and dark circles are a concern. Adding one to your routine may help your eyes look less tired by making those areas appear more even and smooth. Because the skin near the eyes dries out more easily, keeping it properly moisturized throughout the day is important. A lightweight cream that keeps this area soft can help maintain comfort and reduce that tight, dry feeling that sometimes develops during the day.

There's also ongoing support for the use of eye creams to improve how fine lines look around the eyes. With regular use, you will notice the skin feels softer and looks a bit smoother, especially in places where deeper lines are forming. For those with sensitive skin or who wear contact lenses, eye creams are generally a gentle option. Many formulas are made to avoid irritation while still delivering the hydration and care this area often needs.

To apply eye cream, place a small amount on your ring finger, then lightly dab it in tiny dots around the entire eye area during both your morning and evening skincare routines. Gently work it into the skin using upward strokes, making sure to reach the under-eye area, brow bone, outer corners, and even the eyelid, until it fully blends in. Once the cream is absorbed, go ahead with the rest of your routine. Take care not to let any product get into your eyes, and if that happens, rinse thoroughly with water.

Types of Eye Creams

There are several kinds of eye creams, each made to support the delicate skin around the eyes in different ways. Some are designed to help reduce signs of aging, like lines and sagging, while others focus on gently brightening and smoothing the skin using ingredients that encourage surface renewal. There are also options with retinol that work gradually to improve skin texture without being too harsh. For those dealing with dryness, certain creams are made to keep the area well-moisturized throughout the day. And if your skin often feels irritated or tired, soothing formulas are available to bring relief and comfort while supporting a more rested appearance.

Key Difference between Morning vs. Nighttime Routines

Morning and evening skincare routines serve different purposes. What you apply during the day mostly focuses on keeping your skin protected, while your night routine is about helping your skin rest and recover. In the morning, your face may show signs of sleep like puffiness, oiliness, or uneven texture, especially if you've slept on your side or had a rough night. A lack of rest can make your skin look dull, tired, or older than usual. It may even lead to breakouts or irritation. On top of that, your skin faces things like pollution, sunlight, and even the glow from your screen. That's why your morning routine should prepare your skin to face all of it—cleansing to remove any build-up from your pillow or hair, keeping it moisturized throughout the day, and using products that help guard against outside stressors like UV rays or environmental debris.

As for the evening, your skin shifts into recovery mode. After a full day of exposure to sun and pollutants, it's important to support its natural repair process. At night, your routine should aim to refresh your skin, address any concerns, and help it lock in moisture so it can recover overnight. This is the time to add products that help soften the look of blemishes or dryness and maintain a smooth and even texture. When using different products, the way you apply them matters. If you layer products the wrong way, your skin might not absorb them as well. The general rule is to apply from lightest to heaviest. Start with water-based products like toner or essences and work your way up to creams and oils. If your routine includes vitamin C for brightness, hyaluronic acid for moisture, or retinol for fine lines, make sure you use them in the right order for the best results. Sunscreen should always be the final layer in your daytime routine, and the only things that go over it are your makeup products like foundation or powder. Including an essence after cleansing is also helpful. This step softens the skin and can help it better take in whatever you apply next, making your overall routine more effective without being too harsh.

Chapter Five

Seasonal Adjustments to Your Routine

Winter Skincare Routine

As the weather shifts and cooler temperatures roll in, it's not unusual to notice that your skin feels drier than usual. Some people respond to this by overhauling their entire skincare routine, but that isn't always necessary. Your skin type remains the same—what changes is the need for extra comfort and moisture. Making a few small tweaks, like switching to richer products or adding something soothing, can be all you need to keep your skin feeling good during winter.

Cold air, low humidity, and strong winds tend to pull water from your skin, and indoor heating doesn't help—it only adds to the dryness. These seasonal elements can leave your face feeling tight, looking red, or feeling rough to the touch. Even those with oily or mixed skin types aren't immune. During this time of year, sensitivity and water loss are common across the board.

The reason your skin may feel rough or flaky in the colder months often comes down to the contrast between outdoor chill and the warm air pumped through homes and buildings. Hot showers can also make things worse by removing the skin's natural oils. Signs of seasonal dryness often include flaking, itching, dullness, and that familiar tight feeling after cleansing.

There's no need to start from scratch when the season changes. Instead, try using a heavier moisturizer, switching to a more soothing cleanser, or adding a product designed to support skin that's struggling with dryness. These simple swaps can make a big difference and help you maintain a smooth, soft surface.

Daily moisturizing is key. For dry or normal skin, rich creams or ointments do better than lighter options. If you have sensitive skin, stick to fragrance-free formulas that don't include lanolin. It's best to apply your moisturizer while your skin is still damp after washing to help hold on to moisture.

Be careful not to over-wash your skin. Over-cleansing can strip it of its natural oils. You only need to focus on cleaning your face, hands, feet, and areas that crease once a day. For the rest of your body, plain water or minimal product use is often enough.

It's also smart to limit hot water and harsh soaps. If you're dealing with itchy or dry patches, shorter, warm baths or showers with a gentle, soap-free cleanser can help. After bathing, apply a thick cream or ointment to lock in hydration and avoid scrubbing your skin too hard.

Using a humidifier can bring some much-needed moisture back into your indoor space, which your skin will thank you for. Just remember to keep the device clean and follow the care instructions to prevent buildup of unwanted substances. When you're outdoors, cover your face when possible, and protect your lips with something rich like a balm. Formulas that include ceramides or thicker ointments offer good support. Try not to expose yourself to extreme cold for long periods, as it can trigger discomfort or more serious skin issues. If you notice pain, discoloration, or numbness in your fingers or toes, especially with sores or blisters, don't ignore it—speak with a doctor.

Even though it might feel gloomy outside, winter sun can still harm your skin. If you're going to be outside for any length of time, apply a product with at least SPF 15. Sun damage doesn't take a break just because it's cold. Skip tanning beds, too. They're not safer in winter and carry the same risks year-round. If you like a bit of color, self-tanning lotions with added moisture can give you a glow without drying your skin out.

Because you're getting less sunshine, your body may not produce as much vitamin D as it does during summer. Taking a supplement can help maintain healthy levels through the colder months. For an extra boost, try adding a rich, calming face mask once in a while, especially when the weather is particularly harsh. A mask made with avocado, for instance, can help refresh tired-looking skin and bring back softness.

Before bed, take advantage of the fact that your skin is more ready to absorb moisture. A thick night cream or soothing serum can work well while you sleep, helping to restore hydration overnight. If you're dealing with skin that doesn't seem to improve or you're noticing rashes, scaling, or other uncomfortable changes, don't wait—book a visit with your dermatologist. Winter may be rough on skin, but with a few smart habits, you can get through it comfortably.

Look for ingredients that are known to help during colder weather. These include squalane, ceramides, hyaluronic acid, glycerin, and avocado oil. They each play a part in keeping your skin feeling soft, calm, and protected when the air outside isn't on your side.

Summer Skincare Routine

As the warmer months roll in, filled with sunshine and more time spent outdoors, it becomes important to shift your skincare habits to better suit the challenges brought by the season. The summer heat, along with higher humidity and increased exposure to the sun, means your skin will likely need different kinds of support than it does during cooler months.

To start, you'll want to include a cleanser that keeps your face clean without removing the natural oils that keep your skin feeling comfortable. Use it morning and night to help wash away buildup from sweat, dirt, and outdoor exposure. After cleansing, a toner can help clear away any leftover impurities and reduce the look of large pores. Choose one that is gentle and non-drying, and apply it with a soft cotton pad. Following your toner, reach for a lightweight serum that targets whatever your skin might need—hydration, brightness, or added smoothness. A water-based moisturizer comes next, ideally one that keeps your skin soft without leaving it greasy or clogging pores. This is especially helpful for those with oilier skin or who are prone to breakouts during the summer.

No summer routine is complete without proper sun protection. Choose a broad-spectrum sunscreen with an SPF of at least 30. Apply it generously and don't forget to reapply every couple of hours, especially after sweating or being in the water. Keeping your lips covered with a balm that includes sun protection is just as important, since they're easily affected by sun and wind. Drinking enough water throughout the day also plays a part in how your skin behaves in the heat. Staying hydrated helps your body function well and supports skin that feels less tight and looks more refreshed. Pair this with food that's rich in fruits, vegetables, and good fats to keep your skin clear and balanced from the inside out.

You may also want to take cooler showers, especially after a long day outdoors. Hot water can strip your skin, so lukewarm or cool water helps maintain moisture. After bathing, gently pat your skin dry and apply your moisturizer while your skin is still slightly damp. Try to avoid heavy makeup during summer days. Thicker products can block your pores and lead to blemishes. A tinted moisturizer or light foundation is a better choice when it's hot outside. It's also smart to get enough sleep every night, which allows your skin to recover from the day's exposure to sun and heat.

If you're spending time outside, wear a hat and clothes that cover more of your skin. Lightweight, breathable fabrics can keep you comfortable while offering another layer of protection. Sunglasses that block both UVA and UVB rays will help protect the sensitive skin around your eyes too. When possible, stay out of the sun between mid-morning and late afternoon, as this is when UV rays are strongest. If you do need to be out during that time, take breaks in the shade and remember to refresh your sunscreen.

Adding a nourishing mask once in a while can give your skin an extra boost when it feels tired or dry. A formula with ingredients like avocado oil can be especially comforting. And during sleep, your skin is more receptive to moisture, so applying a night cream or serum before bed helps lock in hydration while your body rests.

If you notice unusual dryness, breakouts, or anything concerning, don't hesitate to check in with a skin specialist. Making these simple adjustments can help keep your skin calm, balanced, and comfortable all season long.

Transitioning Between Seasons

When the seasons shift, your skincare routine should shift too. One of the most effective ways to manage this is by adjusting your moisturizer depending on the weather—lighter, fast-absorbing products during warmer months, and richer creams once the air turns cold and dry. As spring comes around, gentle exfoliation can help sweep away any rough patches left by winter. No matter the season, one thing remains constant: proper sun protection. Always use sunscreen that meets your needs, even on cloudy days.

Cleansers are another part of your routine worth reviewing. As the weather changes, consider using a formula that gives your skin more hydration or is better suited for sensitivity. Taking care of your skin through each part of the year means noticing how it reacts to shifts in temperature, wind, humidity, and sunlight. Our skin, being the body's largest protective layer, often mirrors the environment around us. Just like you change your clothes, hobbies, or favorite meals depending on the season, your skincare approach deserves that same attention. Supporting your skin with the right products and care throughout the year helps keep it feeling smooth, strong, and comfortable.

Depending on your location, you may already be feeling the effects of warmer weather, or you might still be waiting for the chill to pass. For instance, spring has started in Southern Finland, but the nights are still cold and the lakes haven't quite thawed. Even though it still feels like winter, there's something exciting about the coming of May and everything it brings. As the months change, some tweaks to your routine can make a big difference. In spring, it's helpful to lightly buff away dead skin and brighten your tone. You might also want to give your SPF a second look and consider something stronger. It's also a good time to pay attention to any skin changes, such as new or changing moles. Products with vitamin C and other protective ingredients can be a great addition during this season. If your skin needs both oil and water-based care, layering your products with intention can help keep things balanced.

When the cooler winds of fall start to move in, it's worth focusing more on moisture. Adding richer formulas and body care like hand creams and balms can help with the dryness that tends to come with the season. As daylight shortens, it may be the right time to start using stronger treatments, especially those that aren't recommended with too much sun exposure. Gentle exfoliation still has its place here, and so do deeply moisturizing steps that support your skin barrier.

In summer, it's best to avoid heavy creams that can clog pores or feel uncomfortable in the heat. Instead, stick with light, water-based lotions that keep the skin soft without feeling greasy. Always use sunscreen—no matter the cloud cover—and wear sun-safe clothing like wide-brimmed hats if you'll be outside. Try not to spend long periods under direct sunlight, especially during peak hours. Hydration is also key, both inside and out. Drinking enough water and using products that help hold moisture in the skin will go a long way. Gentle cleansing is important too, especially after sweating or time outdoors.

Winter tends to be hard on the skin, especially when the air gets cold and heaters run constantly. This combination can lead to tightness, rough patches, and general discomfort. Thicker creams and oil-based balms can help lock in moisture and protect the skin from the dry, biting air. Wearing gloves, scarves, and warm layers helps shield your skin from harsh conditions. Treatments like LED, vitamin A, or microneedling may be more suitable during these months as sun exposure is reduced. It's still important to use sunscreen, even when it's cloudy or snowing. Hot baths may seem tempting, but they can strip the skin of its natural oils, so shorter, lukewarm showers are better.

As autumn returns, think about slowly swapping out your summer skincare for something a bit more nourishing. Introducing hydrating serums and moving toward creamier moisturizers can help your skin transition more smoothly into the colder months. Supporting your skin through each season doesn't require a full overhaul of your routine. Small, thoughtful adjustments that respond to your environment and how your skin feels will make all the difference in how it looks and holds up all year round.

Chapter Six

Skincare Active Ingredients and their functions

Vitamin C: Vitamin C is one of the most widely known and frequently used ingredients in skincare, and for good reason. While many ingredients come and go in popularity, this one has stayed at the top of the list for years. Its reputation is not just about marketing; it has genuine benefits that support both skin appearance and overall skin condition.

This ingredient is most often recommended for its ability to even out the look of skin tone and help defend against environmental stress. It's found in many brightening formulas and is a favorite choice for those looking to improve dullness or uneven texture. But Vitamin C doesn't just help the skin appear more refreshed—it also plays a part in the way the skin naturally repairs itself. It contributes to the process of tissue renewal and supports the skin's ability to stay smooth and firm.

Since the human body can't produce Vitamin C by itself, it needs to be taken in from outside sources. That includes what we eat, supplements we take, and products we apply to the skin. In skincare, this ingredient appears in many forms. The most recognized and direct type is L-Ascorbic Acid, but you'll also see names like Magnesium Ascorbyl Phosphate, Sodium Ascorbyl Phosphate, Ascorbyl Palmitate, and Ethyl Ascorbic Acid. These versions exist because pure Vitamin C can be quite unstable. It reacts easily when exposed to air, heat, water, or other substances, which can weaken its performance and cause it to break down too quickly.

To work around this, skincare brands often use these alternative versions that are combined with other ingredients to help preserve the Vitamin C. Once they're applied to the skin, they convert into the active form, giving you the same benefits in a more lasting and manageable way. This is also why many Vitamin C products, especially serums, come in dark or opaque bottles—to help block light and keep the formula stable for as long as possible. If your Vitamin C serum starts to turn brown, that's a sign the formula has started to lose its strength, and it's best to stop using it.

Retinol: Retinol is a well-known form of Vitamin A, widely recognized in skincare for helping improve the look of aging skin. It's part of a group known as retinoids, which includes both over-the-counter and prescription-strength options. What sets retinol apart is its availability in milder concentrations, making it a common ingredient in cosmetic products aimed at smoothing fine lines, improving texture and supporting overall skin renewal.

This ingredient works by connecting with certain receptors in the skin, which triggers quicker cell turnover. It also helps slow the breakdown of collagen, a protein that keeps skin firm. Although prescription-strength retinoids are stronger and deliver faster results, they also carry a higher risk of irritation. In comparison, retinol products found in drugstores or beauty retailers work more gradually and are better suited for those easing into this part of their skincare routine.

In Canada, for example, many top-tier skincare products contain between 0.3% to 1% retinol, which is enough to be effective while still being gentle for most users. Prescription versions, which include higher percentages, are typically reserved for specific skin concerns and require professional supervision. When starting out, it's recommended to begin with a lower percentage and increase only if your skin responds well. This helps avoid discomfort like redness, dryness, or flaking, which are common when using stronger formulas too soon.

There are several versions of retinoids that you may come across. One of the mildest is Retinyl Palmitate, often suggested for those with dry or easily irritated skin. Slightly stronger is Retinaldehyde, another non-prescription option. Retinol itself is one of the most popular and potent versions you can buy without a prescription. Tretinoin and Tazarotene, on the other hand, are only available through a doctor and are typically used for more targeted treatment.

Many retinol products come blended with ingredients like moisturizers or calming agents. These additions help reduce the chance of irritation and support better results, but they can also affect how much retinol actually reaches your skin. That's one of the reasons why creating a stable retinol formula is a challenge. It's not just about the amount—it's also about how well the product holds up over time and under different storage conditions. To help protect the formula, brands often package retinol in containers that keep air and light out. This preserves its strength and keeps the product working as intended.

Hyaluronic acid: Hyaluronic acid is a naturally occurring compound found in the body's connective tissues, particularly in the skin. It belongs to a group of long-chain sugar molecules known as glycolsaminoglycans, which play a key role in keeping the skin looking full and hydrated. While collagen is associated with skincare, hyaluronic acid is just as important. It supports the skin's framework and is one of the main reasons youthful skin feels so supple. Over time, the body's natural supply decreases, which can lead to more visible lines, dryness, and a loss of firmness.

This ingredient has gained popularity for good reason. One of its most impressive traits is its ability to retain water—up to 1,000 times its own weight. That means it acts like a magnet for moisture, helping the skin stay hydrated and soft. When people talk about skin looking fresh or feeling smooth, it often comes down to how much water is present in the surface layers. That's where hyaluronic acid makes a difference. It binds water to the skin and slows the natural loss of moisture that happens throughout the day.

The term "trans-epidermal water loss," or TEWL, refers to how much water evaporates from the skin. Products that help reduce TEWL work by keeping hydration where it's needed—within the skin layers. Hyaluronic acid plays a big role in this process, acting like a barrier that holds moisture in and keeps dryness at bay. Because of this, it's a great addition to routines aimed at maintaining a healthy, dewy look.

Besides locking in moisture, hyaluronic acid has also been studied for its ability to support skin recovery. It has a calming effect on irritated areas and may help reduce redness and surface discomfort. That's why it's often used in products that soothe or protect the skin. For people dealing with dryness, sensitivity, or aging-related concerns, this ingredient offers a gentle yet effective option to keep the skin balanced and well cared for.

Its structure allows it to absorb and hold water while working with other components in the skin to keep everything functioning smoothly. It's no surprise that hyaluronic acid has become a trusted ingredient across a wide range of skincare products, from serums to moisturizers. Whether someone is looking to improve hydration or simply keep their skin comfortable throughout the day, this ingredient is a reliable choice that fits into nearly any routine.

Niacinamide: Niacinamide, also known as vitamin B3 or nicotinamide, is a versatile ingredient that plays a valuable role in skincare. Found in trace amounts in foods like meat, wheat, and fish, the version used in beauty products is made in labs and refined for topical use. It's a water-soluble vitamin that appears as a fine white powder, free of scent and with a slightly bitter taste, though taste doesn't matter much when it comes to applying it to your face. What does matter is how much it can do for your skin. This vitamin has become a favorite in many skincare routines because it offers a wide range of benefits without being harsh or irritating. Whether your concerns are oiliness, dryness, uneven tone, or general skin clarity, niacinamide can step in and help restore balance. It's gentle enough for regular use but effective enough to make a visible difference over time.

One of its key strengths is how it supports the skin's barrier. This means it helps the outer layer of the skin stay strong and hold on to moisture, which is especially important for keeping your face looking and feeling smooth. At the same time, it can help reduce the appearance of dark spots, improve tone, and even out areas that may be affected by past breakouts or sun exposure.

For those dealing with redness or irritation, niacinamide brings a calming touch. It can help minimize flare-ups and soothe discomfort without clogging pores or leaving behind residue. People with oily or acne-prone skin often find it helpful, as it can reduce excess shine and keep pores clearer with regular use. Aside from all that, it gives the skin a more refined texture and a healthier-looking surface. It doesn't work like a quick fix, but with consistent use, it helps your skin stay on track—fewer breakouts, a more even tone, and a smoother feel overall. It's no surprise that some people consider this ingredient a go-to for keeping their skincare simple yet effective. Whether used in serums, moisturizers, or toners, niacinamide easily fits into daily routines and quietly works to bring out the best in your skin.

AHA and BHA: AHAs and BHAs are two commonly used types of hydroxy acids in skincare that support the skin's natural exfoliation process. They help shed old, dull skin cells and bring out smoother, clearer, more even skin underneath. Though these ingredients might sound technical, they've been part of skincare routines for generations.

In fact, historical accounts suggest that Cleopatra used to bathe in sour milk, which naturally contains lactic acid, a type of AHA, to improve her skin's softness and tone. Today, these acids show up in everything from facial washes to body lotions and toners, making them easily accessible to anyone interested in skincare.

AHAs, or alpha-hydroxy acids, are water-based acids often derived from natural sources like fruit, sugarcane, and milk. Though their roots are in nature, most AHAs used in skincare today are produced in labs to ensure consistency and purity. These acids are known for their ability to smooth out the skin's surface by gently breaking down the bonds between dead skin cells, allowing them to be washed away more easily. AHAs have become especially popular in products designed to target signs of sun exposure, discoloration, or aging skin, and are often included in creams, serums, and exfoliators.

BHAs, or beta-hydroxy acids, are another group of exfoliating acids that are oil-soluble. This makes them especially helpful for people with oily or acne-prone skin, as they can reach deeper into pores and remove built-up oil and debris. BHAs also come from natural sources, like willow bark, but they're typically made in labs for skincare use. One of the most common BHAs is salicylic acid, a familiar ingredient to many dealing with clogged pores or uneven skin texture.

While both AHAs and BHAs clear away dead skin cells, they work in different ways. AHAs stay on the surface and are ideal for targeting issues like dullness, dry patches, and early signs of aging. BHAs, on the other hand, can travel into the pores and clear out oil, making them better for blemishes and congestion. BHAs tend to be gentler on the skin due to their larger molecular size, which means they don't penetrate as quickly as AHAs like glycolic acid. Because of this, some people may find AHAs slightly more likely to cause sensitivity or redness, especially if used in higher concentrations or too frequently.

AHAs contribute to smoother texture and support natural turnover by softening the outer layer of the skin. This helps reduce surface lines, brighten tone, and keep moisture in by exposing fresher, more hydrated skin cells. They're also useful for people who want to reduce the appearance of acne marks, dry patches, or uneven tone. BHAs, thanks to their oil-loving nature, can deeply cleanse the pores, helping to calm breakouts, clean out blackheads, and smooth out rough texture on oily skin.

To find out if a product contains either of these acids, it's helpful to check the ingredient list. For AHAs, look for words like glycolic acid, lactic acid, citric acid, or hydroxycaprylic acid. If it's a BHA, you might see salicylic acid or other names like willow bark extract, sodium salicylate, or tropic acid. Some skincare products even include both types, offering a combination that works across different layers of the skin.

Peptides: Peptides have become a familiar word in skincare conversations, often praised for their impressive effects on the skin. But what exactly are they, and why are they considered so useful in personal care products? Peptides are short chains made from amino acids—the same building blocks that form proteins. In skincare, these tiny molecules play a big role in supporting the skin's structure and overall condition. Collagen, elastin, and keratin are all proteins that help keep the skin smooth, strong, and youthful, and peptides can encourage their production when applied to the skin.

Applying peptides through skincare can help the skin produce more of the proteins it needs to stay firm and flexible. This can lead to a more lifted appearance and a smoother texture. There are different types of peptides, and each has its own function. Some help carry minerals like copper or magnesium to the skin, supporting healing and enzyme processes. Others help block the action of enzymes that break down collagen, which can help the skin stay more elastic over time. Certain kinds, called neuropeptides, can even interrupt signals that cause muscles to contract, which may lead to fewer expression lines.

One of the main reasons peptides are used in skincare is their ability to support collagen production. Collagen helps the skin stay firm and resist sagging. As we age, collagen production slows down, which leads to the formation of fine lines and wrinkles. By stimulating collagen, peptides can help give the skin a more youthful look. They also support the skin's outer barrier, which plays a role in keeping moisture in and irritants out. A strong barrier means better hydration and overall smoother texture.

These ingredients can also play a part in reducing redness or discomfort. Their support in forming collagen and elastin helps maintain firmness, while their calming properties can be useful after treatments or for skin that's healing. Some peptides even help soften the appearance of wrinkles by limiting muscle movement in a way that's often compared to popular injectables. Incorporating peptides into your daily routine can be simple. While cleansers containing peptides may not stay on the skin long enough to bring lasting results, they can still help keep skin soft and hydrated during use. For deeper benefits, applying a peptide-based serum after cleansing and before your moisturizer allows better absorption. Many serums focus on delivering a strong amount of peptides to encourage skin renewal and strength.

There are several categories of peptides used in skincare, and each plays a unique part. Some help block enzymes, others send signals to start cell repair, and a few deliver minerals where they're needed. Peptides like Matrixyl—often listed as palmitoyl- or oligopeptide pentapeptide—are found in many creams and serums aimed at smoothing fine lines. Palmitoyl oligopeptide is known for prompting the skin to make more collagen and elastin. If pigmentation is a concern, oligopeptide-8 helps slow the process that causes dark patches or melasma. Acetyl hexapeptide-3 works in a way similar to injectables that relax muscle movement, softening expression lines without the need for a needle.

Chapter Seven

Natural and Synthetic Ingredients

The packaging draws you in, the scent feels calming, and the idea of using something straight from nature seems like the safest route for your skin. It's easy to assume that choosing "natural" skincare means you're giving your skin something pure and safe. But that's not always true. Terms like "natural" and "clean" are not officially regulated, which means brands can use them freely without needing to meet any fixed guidelines. And while plant-based ingredients can sound gentle, they aren't always friendly to sensitive skin. In fact, they can be a major cause of skin reactions. The term "natural" generally refers to ingredients that are sourced from plants or other elements found in nature rather than those created in a lab. But this definition is loose. Just because something comes from a plant doesn't mean it's good for your face—plenty of plants in the wild can cause serious skin irritation. The lack of a clear definition means that a product labeled "natural" might still contain ingredients that could bother your skin, especially if you're prone to sensitivity.

In the United States, there is no strict rule from the Food and Drug Administration that defines what can or cannot be marketed as natural skincare. That creates a gray area where almost anything can be labeled in a way that gives the impression it's safer or gentler than it actually is. And while natural oils, extracts, and minerals can bring benefits to the skin, they can also lead to problems. A product might be filled with botanical ingredients and still cause redness, breakouts, or itchiness in people who don't even realize they have a sensitivity to those components. Believing that this kind of reaction is rare is a mistake. One study from 2023 reviewed around 1,700 skincare products marketed as natural, clean, or sensitive skin-friendly. Shockingly, more than 94% of them contained ingredients that have been linked to contact dermatitis, a condition where the skin becomes red, inflamed, and uncomfortable. The exact symptoms these products promise to prevent can end up being caused by the very ingredients they contain.

So while it's tempting to trust a product just because it carries a "natural" label, the reality is more complicated. Choosing skincare should be about how your skin responds to an ingredient, not just where that ingredient comes from. The best product for your skin might come from a lab, a plant, or both—it all depends on what works for you.

Understanding Synthetic Skincare Ingredients

Synthetic skincare refers to products made using lab-created ingredients, many of which are developed to mimic or improve upon what's found in nature. These ingredients often start out from natural sources but go through chemical processes to become more refined and effective. While some substances like phthalates, silicones, and parabens are often talked about negatively, not every lab-made ingredient deserves the same reaction. Many, including hyaluronic acid and retinol, are widely accepted and praised for their results. There's a belief that natural ingredients are better for the skin, but this isn't always the case. Some natural extracts can clog pores or trigger breakouts, especially when they don't match a person's skin type. On the flip side, certain synthetic compounds are known to deliver moisture or target signs of aging more effectively without the same risk of irritation.

One of the reasons synthetic ingredients can be preferable is their consistency. In a controlled environment, scientists can measure and balance ingredients precisely, leading to a more stable formula. This reduces the likelihood of variation from batch to batch and often extends the shelf life of the product. That's an advantage when compared to many natural ingredients, which may degrade faster or behave unpredictably. Another factor to consider is that many synthetic ingredients have gone through rigorous testing for performance and skin compatibility. In contrast, some natural substances are used without extensive review and can lead to irritation or allergic reactions. Lab-made formulas can be just as effective—or even better—than those using only plants and minerals. Their performance depends largely on how they're formulated and the strength of the active ingredients. Some of the most dependable synthetic ingredients are used to improve moisture, reduce breakouts, or firm the skin. Many versions are also made to resemble the structure of natural elements already found in the body, allowing them to work smoothly without causing harm.

That said, synthetic skincare isn't without concerns. Certain ingredients can lead to clogged pores or sensitivity, just as natural ones can. And from an environmental standpoint, making synthetic ingredients often requires energy and resources. However, relying on lab-made versions can also help reduce overharvesting of plant species, making it a more responsible choice in some situations. Marketing can complicate matters further. Products labeled as "eco-friendly" or "natural" often come with imagery that suggests purity and sustainability, even when that's not truly reflected in the formula. This is called greenwashing, and it's common in the beauty world. Brands may use earthy colors, floral graphics, or vague terms like "clean" to give an impression of being safer or better for the planet. But without specific details or clear certification, it's hard to tell what's actually in the bottle.

Sometimes, these products list only a few plant-based ingredients and still contain synthetic additives or chemicals that aren't as skin-friendly. Even claims like "paraben-free" or "sulfate-free" can be misleading if the alternatives used aren't well understood or have similar drawbacks. Scents labeled as "natural" may still contain artificial elements, and just because packaging looks biodegradable or recycled doesn't mean the formula inside is made with the same care.

If you're trying to make informed choices, it's better to check the full ingredient list than to rely on marketing language. Be cautious of products that boast high percentages of natural ingredients without explaining how those numbers are calculated. In some cases, water is included in that figure to make it sound more impressive than it actually is. Products that don't clearly disclose all their ingredients or how those ingredients were sourced should also raise questions. And if the names on the label are difficult to read or sound overly technical, it's worth doing a bit more research. Compounds like sodium lauryl sulfate, PEGs, dimethicone, or tetrasodium can show up in products that seem natural at first glance, but may not be ideal for your skin or the environment.

Chapter Eight

Ingredients to Avoid

Alcohol often sneaks into skincare products more than most people realize. While it can make formulas feel lightweight, quick-drying, or refreshing, not all types of alcohol are equally kind to your skin. It's easy to be misled by confusing information floating around online, but when you take a closer look at the evidence, it becomes clear that some forms of alcohol—especially when high on an ingredient list—can do more harm than good. These are the kinds that strip away the skin's natural balance, interfere with its ability to bounce back, and weaken its outer layers. Before tossing everything in your cabinet labeled with the word "alcohol," it's worth knowing which kinds should raise a red flag and which can actually support your skincare routine.

The troublemakers usually appear under names like denatured alcohol, isopropyl alcohol, or SD alcohol. These are used to thin out products and leave a non-greasy finish, which appeals especially to those with oily or acne-prone skin. While they may give that instant clean or matte look, they do so by drying out the skin, breaking down its barrier, and eventually triggering even more oil production. Over time, instead of balancing the skin, these ingredients can lead to roughness, enlarged pores, and irritation. When such alcohols show up among the top ingredients in a product, they're doing more than just a little surface drying—they're disrupting the skin's natural defenses. On the other hand, there are types of alcohol known as fatty alcohols that are quite different. These include ingredients like cetyl alcohol, cetearyl alcohol, and stearyl alcohol. Despite having "alcohol" in the name, they don't act in the same way as the harsh ones. Fatty alcohols are often added to products for their creamy texture and ability to lock in moisture. They can help improve consistency, make products feel richer, and support dry or sensitive skin without causing irritation. These are not only safe but beneficial when used appropriately.

There's also a common claim that alcohol helps other ingredients—like vitamin C or retinol—penetrate deeper into the skin. While this has some truth, the side effects of using harsh alcohols can undo the good those ingredients are meant to deliver. Thankfully, there are gentler ways to help products absorb without damaging the skin's natural surface. People with oily or breakout-prone skin often gravitate toward products with drying alcohols because they seem to reduce shine right away. But what happens next isn't so helpful. These alcohols strip away natural oils and irritate the skin, which can trigger more oil production and breakouts. In the long run, this just keeps the cycle going. It's a short-term fix that creates long-term setbacks.

Scientific findings consistently show that the wrong types of alcohol can weaken the skin's surface, wash away key substances the skin needs to stay strong, and worsen existing skin concerns. Choosing products that rely on these alcohols when better options exist simply doesn't make sense anymore—especially when there are so many gentler, more nourishing ingredients available.

There is, however, one major exception where strong alcohol is not only acceptable but necessary—hand sanitizer. When washing with soap and water isn't an option, sanitizers with at least 60% alcohol help eliminate harmful bacteria and viruses. Although regular exposure to these products may dry out your hands, the benefit in this case outweighs the drawback. Just be sure to follow up with a moisturizer to help your hands recover. So, while alcohol in skincare might seem harmless or even helpful at first, the reality is that many forms can be far from friendly to your skin's long-term health. It's worth paying close attention to the ingredient list and opting for products that support your skin without compromising its natural balance.

Fragrance: Yay or Nay?

Fragrance shows up in all kinds of skincare—foundations, cleansers, serums, moisturizers. While these scents can make a product more appealing to use, the same can't always be said for how they affect your skin. Whether the source is synthetic or from a flower or essential oil, fragrance in skincare is one of the most common reasons people experience skin trouble.

The assumption is that if an ingredient is natural, it must be safe. That's not always true. Natural fragrance can be just as harsh on your skin as synthetic fragrance. In fact, both types can cause reactions, especially if your skin is already on the sensitive side. Even if you don't consider your skin to be delicate or reactive, that doesn't mean fragranced products are doing you any favors. Repeated use, even without obvious redness or stinging, can still affect your skin's balance. You may not notice the impact right away, but small amounts of irritation build up over time. This may show later in the form of uneven tone, dryness, or even fine lines. According to the American Academy of Dermatology, fragrance is the leading cause of allergic reactions linked to cosmetics. You might already know how uncomfortable irritated skin feels if you've ever overused retinol or a strong acid—it's that hot, itchy, sensitive sensation that seems impossible to calm. While fragrance doesn't always cause an immediate response, it can still spark inflammation beneath the surface. Just because you don't see red patches or breakouts doesn't mean it's harmless. The changes it causes may take time to appear, much like how sun damage shows up years after repeated exposure without sunscreen.

It's easy to wonder why brands would still include fragrance if it can lead to these issues. The answer is surprisingly simple: consumers are drawn to products that not only perform well but also feel and smell good. A product can work wonders for the skin, but if it smells unpleasant or clinical, people are less likely to keep using it. Scent helps create a pleasant experience, even if it comes at a cost to your skin's long-term condition.

So how do you know if your skincare includes fragrance that might be doing more harm than good? The key is to check the ingredient list. Look for terms like "fragrance" or "parfum," which usually indicate added scent. You'll also want to be cautious with certain essential oils. While they may sound gentle or plant-based, oils such as lavender, rose, orange, eucalyptus, and geranium can be irritating for some people. Just because something smells good doesn't mean your skin will tolerate it. Some ingredients like vanilla or almond might have a sweet scent and pose little risk, so it's not always about the fragrance itself but the source and concentration. Other names to watch out for include linalool, limonene, eugenol, citronellol, and cinnamal—common irritants found in scented skincare. If you're unsure whether a product is triggering your skin issues, it's a good idea to patch test before applying it to your face. Dab a small amount behind your ear or on your inner arm and wait a full day to see if your skin reacts. If no itching, redness, or bumps appear, the product may be safe to use more broadly.

At the end of the day, even if your skin seems fine now, repeated exposure to irritating ingredients can gradually wear down its defenses. Being more selective with what you put on your skin can help you avoid problems before they start.

Harsh Preservatives and Parabens

Parabens are a group of synthetic ingredients that have been widely used as preservatives in beauty and personal care products since the early 20th century. These chemicals are added to prevent the growth of harmful bacteria and mold, helping products stay safe and last longer on the shelf. While their role in extending product life is well known, concerns have grown over how they interact with the body. Scientific findings suggest that parabens may disrupt the body's hormone system. This interference could affect fertility and the function of reproductive organs. Some studies also point to potential effects on birth health and even link long-term exposure to a greater risk of developing certain types of cancer. In addition, parabens may cause reactions in the skin, particularly in sensitive individuals.

Research carried out in the United States has detected parabens in nearly all urine samples collected from adults, regardless of background or lifestyle. This widespread exposure highlights how common these compounds are in everyday products. Specific types, like isobutylparaben, butylparaben, isopropylparaben and propylparaben, are of particular concern due to their stronger impact on the hormone system and their possible connection to reproductive problems in both men and women. What's clear is that daily use of products containing these types of parabens may lead to repeated exposure over a lifetime. Considering the health concerns they raise, it's worth noting that many companies have already started creating formulas without them. Skincare and beauty products can be made just as effective without including these ingredients, offering safer choices for those who want to reduce their exposure.

Types of Parabens

Parabens have been part of cosmetic and skincare product formulas since the 1920s. These ingredients are commonly listed on product labels, especially on items like shampoos, conditioners, lotions, and makeup. When scanning the ingredients list, you might come across names such as methylparaben, ethylparaben, propylparaben, isopropylparaben, butylparaben, and isobutylparaben. It's not unusual for more than one of these to appear in the same product. Manufacturers often combine different types to increase the effectiveness of preservation and extend shelf life, especially in products that contain water or other ingredients prone to bacterial growth.

Parabens are still found in many personal care items used daily. In your home, you might come across them in products such as shampoos, conditioners, and other hair treatments. They also appear in moisturizers, face creams, and a wide range of makeup items. Shaving products can contain them too. In the past, they were often included in deodorants and antiperspirants, although many companies have now reformulated to leave them out. Despite growing awareness, some brands still rely on these ingredients, so it's important to read product labels if you're trying to avoid them.

Why you should Avoid Parabens based products

Most people choose to stay away from parabens in their skincare products due to concerns about how these preservatives might interact with the body. One of the biggest concerns is that parabens can imitate estrogen, a hormone that plays a key role in the body. This has raised questions about the possibility of hormone imbalance, and some researchers have looked into whether long-term exposure could be linked to conditions like breast cancer. While findings remain under review and not all studies agree, the uncertainty has led many to opt for products that don't include these ingredients. For some people, parabens can cause skin reactions, though this is less common. Even though certain health authorities consider them acceptable for use, growing caution among users has encouraged many brands to create alternatives without these additives.

In addition to parabens, there are other artificial preservatives that raise concern. Ingredients like BHT, sulfites, BHA, formaldehyde, nitrates, and certain benzoates are sometimes included in formulas to extend shelf life. However, frequent exposure to these can be linked to skin irritation, hormonal changes, and other health concerns. For those looking to avoid such risks, it's worth reading product labels and choosing gentler options when possible.

Skincare During Pregnancy

During pregnancy, it's important to be careful about what goes onto your skin, as certain ingredients can affect not just you but your baby too. Some products are considered safe and can help manage common skin concerns like breakouts or dullness that may arise due to hormonal changes.

Ingredients that are generally considered safe include alpha hydroxy acids such as glycolic and lactic acid. These help gently exfoliate the skin and improve texture. Azelaic acid is another option that helps with redness and acne. Benzoyl peroxide, when used in small amounts, may be considered okay as well, though it's always smart to check with your healthcare provider. Salicylic acid, citric acid, hydroxyacetic acid, and similar types may be used in low concentrations and under guidance. These ingredients help with exfoliation, oil control, and keeping the skin clear. Lactic acid and 2-hydroxyethanoic acid are also among the common ingredients that many consider mild and usable during this period.

On the other hand, there are some components you should avoid while expecting. Retinoids—commonly found in many anti-aging products—fall into this category. This includes products labeled with names like tretinoin, retinol, retinoic acid, and retinyl palmitate, among others. Prescription-strength formulas such as Tazorac (tazarotene), Avita, and Differin should also be left out of your routine for now. These ingredients are known for their powerful cell turnover effects but have been linked to potential risks during pregnancy.

If you're unsure about any product or ingredient, it's a good idea to ask your doctor before using it. Skincare doesn't have to be complicated during pregnancy, but being informed helps you make safer choices for you and your baby.

Chapter Nine

Age-based Skincare Routine

Skincare for Teens

Managing Teenage Acne: Taking care of teenage acne requires a steady and simple routine that focuses on keeping the skin clean and reducing excess oil. Using gentle products that don't contain heavy oils is a good place to start. Look for face washes that are light on the skin and free from ingredients that may clog pores. Washing the face twice a day with lukewarm water and a mild cleanser helps remove buildup from the day.

To manage breakouts, consider using non-prescription treatments that contain ingredients like benzoyl peroxide or salicylic acid. These can help minimize spots and keep future ones from forming. Be sure to apply these only where needed, as using too much can cause dryness or irritation. Makeup can also play a part. Try using products labeled as non-comedogenic, meaning they are less likely to block pores. It's also important to remove makeup fully before sleeping to prevent residue from sitting on the skin overnight.

Keeping your hair clean is another helpful step, especially if it tends to be oily or falls across your face. Hair products and natural oils can transfer to the skin, making breakouts more likely. Avoid touching your face during the day. Our hands come into contact with many surfaces, and transferring bacteria to the skin can worsen acne. If the breakouts are severe or don't improve, it may be time to see a dermatologist for treatment tailored to your skin's needs. Consistency and patience are key when caring for teenage skin.

Building a Simple, Effective Routine

A reliable skincare routine, both in the morning and at night, goes beyond simply washing your face. It's about taking steps to keep your skin nourished, balanced, and protected throughout the day and while you sleep. At the very least, your daily routine should include a gentle cleanser to remove dirt or buildup, a moisturizer to maintain hydration, and sunscreen to guard against sun damage.

Depending on your skin's needs, you can build on this foundation by adding specific treatments. For example, if you're dealing with dryness, choose a moisturizer with added hydration support. If breakouts are a concern, include a product designed to clear pores or calm irritation. Those with oil-prone skin may benefit from lightweight formulas that help manage shine, while products that support smoother texture or firmness can be useful for those focused on aging.

Keeping it simple helps you stay consistent, and tailoring your approach to what your skin responds to is what makes a routine effective over time.

Morning Skincare Routine

A morning skincare routine sets the tone for your day by clearing away any buildup from the night before and prepping your skin to face the elements. It's also a great way to keep your skin hydrated and protected from daily exposure like sunlight and pollution. Start by cleansing your face to remove excess oil and dirt that may clog pores or cause breakouts. Pick a gentle formula without alcohol to avoid drying out your skin. If you're on the dry side, consider using an oil-based cleanser to keep your skin feeling soft. Use lukewarm water and gently massage the cleanser with your fingertips, then rinse and pat your face dry using a soft towel.

When it comes to choosing a cleanser, the right ingredients make a big difference. For dry skin, look for ones that include hyaluronic acid, glycerin, or ceramides. If your skin tends to get oily or break out, try options with ingredients like glycolic acid, salicylic acid, tea tree oil, or benzoyl peroxide. Toner can be used after cleansing, though it's not required for everyone. Depending on the formula, a toner can add moisture or remove leftover oil and impurities. If your skin leans toward dryness or irritation, go for toners with hydrating ingredients like rose water or hyaluronic acid. For those managing oil or acne, toners with salicylic acid or witch hazel are a good match. Apply with a cotton pad or gently tap it onto your face.

If breakouts are a concern, now is the time to apply a targeted acne product or something that helps with dark spots. Use these treatments after cleansing and before moisturizing. You only need a small amount, and it's best to apply them where needed rather than all over unless instructed otherwise. Acne-fighting ingredients such as benzoyl peroxide or salicylic acid can help, while dark spot correctors may include kojic acid or hydroquinone. A serum in the morning can support your skin's brightness, hydration, and protection. Formulas with vitamin C, E, or niacinamide are especially helpful during the day. These antioxidants can help manage damage from sunlight or pollution. Gently press the serum into your face and neck rather than rubbing. If you're using niacinamide, it's best not to combine it with vitamin C at the same time since that can lower its benefits.

Eye cream isn't necessary for everyone, but it can be a helpful step to keep the under-eye area smooth and hydrated. Using your ring finger, lightly tap the product beneath your eyes. During the day, opt for one that includes peptides, vitamin C, or SPF to help reduce puffiness and guard the delicate skin in that area. If you're feeling tired or looking to refresh puffy eyes, caffeine-based formulas may give a more awake appearance. Follow with a moisturizer to lock in hydration. This helps strengthen the skin's outer layer, which protects it from dryness and environmental stress. Even oily skin types benefit from moisturizers to maintain balance and reduce the risk of overproducing oil. Those with dry skin may prefer richer formulas with shea butter, glycerin, or ceramides. If your skin is oily or prone to breakouts, lightweight, gel-based moisturizers with hyaluronic acid work well without clogging pores.

Finally, apply sunscreen. This is the last and one of the most important steps. Sunscreen protects your skin from ultraviolet rays, helping to prevent sunspots, wrinkles, and other damage. Choose a formula labeled broad-spectrum with at least SPF 30. Whether it's sunny or cloudy, indoors or outdoors, apply a nickel-sized amount to your face, neck, ears, and chest. Be sure to reapply every couple of hours if you're spending extended time outside.

Evening Skincare Routine

An evening skincare routine helps wash away the build-up from your day while providing moisture and support for your skin overnight. This process supports skin that might be dry, acne-prone, uneven, or showing signs of aging. Clearing your face before bed allows your skin to breathe and work on healing itself while you sleep.

Start by cleansing your face to remove oils, dirt, and anything else collected throughout the day. You can use the same gentle cleanser from your morning routine, whether it's oil-based or designed to fight breakouts. If you wear makeup, you might need to begin with a separate remover or do a double cleanse to fully clear your skin. Those with oily or acne-prone skin should use micellar water or an oil-free remover to avoid clogging their pores, while people with dry or sensitive skin might benefit from using a balm or oil-based product that both clears makeup and hydrates at the same time.

Toner isn't essential at night, but it can help give your skin a boost by hydrating dry patches or clearing any leftover grime from earlier steps. You might want to switch to an exfoliating toner during your nighttime routine—this can be used once or twice a week to help clean out pores and remove buildup. Those with dry or sensitive skin may prefer something with hyaluronic acid or rose water. For oily skin, salicylic acid or witch hazel may help control oil while you sleep. If your goal is to exfoliate, go for a toner with ingredients like glycolic acid or other AHAs. You can still use spot treatments in the evening to handle breakouts or help fade dark marks. Treatments for pimples usually contain benzoyl peroxide or salicylic acid, while those meant to lighten dark spots may include kojic acid or hydroquinone. Avoid layering too many active ingredients in the same area—alternate them on different nights or apply them to separate parts of the face. If you're treating open pimples, you can also use small healing patches overnight.

Adding a serum or acne treatment across the face in the evening is optional but can be useful, especially if you're working on fine lines or regular breakouts. Stick with just one active ingredient at a time to avoid skin stress. Some nighttime serums gently exfoliate while also moisturizing. For dry skin, look for something with ceramides, vitamin E, peptides, or hyaluronic acid. If you want gentle exfoliation or to smooth rough patches, try glycolic or lactic acid. For acne-prone skin, options with azelaic acid or salicylic acid may help keep pores clear.

Retinol products, which are forms of vitamin A, are another option to consider before bed. They help improve skin texture and support collagen development while reducing clogged pores. These products make your skin more delicate in the sun, so they're best applied at night. If you're trying it for the first time, begin with a small amount every other evening. Those with mild acne or fine lines may choose over-the-counter versions like retinyl palmitate or retinaldehyde. If your skin concerns are more intense, stronger versions such as adapalene or tretinoin may be prescribed by a dermatologist. Some, like Differin, are also available without a prescription. Eye creams at night help refresh the under-eye area and can offer hydration and support for the appearance of fine lines. While not a required step, they're helpful for anyone looking to care for delicate skin. Look for ingredients like niacinamide, retinol, or hyaluronic acid. Keep in mind that retinol can be too strong for some skin types, especially if sensitivity is a concern.

To finish, apply a moisturizer or night cream. These thicker creams are designed to stay in place longer and nourish the skin while you rest. Whether you use your regular moisturizer or something richer, applying one at night keeps your skin from drying out. Choose products with glycerin or hyaluronic acid to add hydration. If you're concerned about breakouts, opt for formulas that are labeled as non-comedogenic, so they won't clog your pores. Some night creams may also contain AHAs or retinol for added support while you sleep.

Facial oils can be an optional final step. They're especially helpful for dry skin and can add another layer of comfort and softness. After your moisturizer, warm a few drops of oil between your hands and press it gently onto your skin. For dry skin, oils like coconut or argan may work well. If your skin is more sensitive, rosehip or chamomile oil can help soothe it. Even if your skin tends to get oily, lightweight oils like jojoba or grapeseed can be used to help manage oil without making your skin feel greasy or blocked.

Additional Tips and Considerations

When putting together a skincare routine, it's a good idea to think about how to introduce or switch products without putting too much pressure on your skin. Being careful with how you layer or rotate treatments can help you avoid irritation or unwanted reactions. It's best not to use alpha hydroxy acids (like glycolic or lactic acid) or beta hydroxy acids (like salicylic acid) at the same time as retinol. If you want to use both in your routine, try using them on different nights. This gives your skin time to adjust and lowers the risk of dryness or sensitivity.

Gentle exfoliation is helpful, but there's no need to do it every day. Many exfoliating products come in the form of toners, cleansers, serums or peels. Using something mild at night is usually fine, but be careful not to pair it with stronger treatments on the same day. Combining multiple exfoliants can be too much and may leave your skin dry or irritated. Face masks are a nice extra step you can take two or three times a week after cleansing and using toner. Depending on the type, they can help balance oily skin or bring moisture to dry areas. Since many masks already contain active ingredients, it's best not to follow them with other treatments, serums or retinol. Instead, finish with a simple moisturizer to help lock in moisture and keep your skin calm.

Skincare in your 20s

In your twenties, your skin often begins to settle into what may become its long-term condition. You might leave behind the unpredictable breakouts of your teenage years, but that doesn't mean you're done with blemishes entirely. Around 3% of adults over 35 still deal with acne, and if your skin leans oily, those breakouts may stick around longer than you'd like. During this decade, it's easy to think your skin can handle anything. Late nights, makeup left on after a long day, or relying on face wipes instead of properly cleansing—it happens. Your skin might bounce back quickly for now, but repeated neglect may catch up with you later.

Taking care of your skin in your twenties isn't just about fixing what you see; it's about setting the stage for what's to come. What you do today matters for how your skin looks and feels in the years ahead. A solid routine now can help you avoid future damage and maintain a smooth, healthy look well into your thirties and beyond. At this age, skincare should focus on keeping your skin clean, well-hydrated and protected. This means using a gentle cleanser, a good moisturizer and daily sun protection. You can also introduce serums and lightweight eye creams to keep your skin fresh and supported without overdoing it. Starting with these basics now can help you maintain a healthy appearance down the road.

Requirement to maintain a healthy skin in my twenties (20s)

Building good habits for your skin during your twenties lays the groundwork for how it will look and feel in the years ahead. At this stage, the main focus should be on protecting against outside elements and making smart choices that support long-term skin strength. While getting older is completely natural and doesn't need to be fought, it's worth noting that collagen—a key part of what keeps skin firm and full—starts to gradually decrease around this time, losing about one percent each year. If you view your skin as a living part of your body, early signs of aging can be seen as a response to damage it's collecting over time. That's why protection matters.

A big part of this includes using sunscreen daily, not just when you're heading to the beach or spending hours outdoors. It's one of the simplest steps you can take to help reduce the impact of both early aging and more serious concerns like skin cancer. Many skip this part of their routine, especially when the weather is cooler or the skies are cloudy, but exposure doesn't stop when the sun isn't visible. It starts from the moment you step outside—and not just from the sun. Light coming from screens, including phones and computers, can also affect your skin. Applying a broad-spectrum sunscreen with at least SPF 30 every morning, even if you're staying inside, helps provide daily protection your skin will thank you for later.

Skincare Routine in my Twenties (20s)

Sticking to a regular skincare routine in your twenties is one of the simplest ways to support healthy skin in the long run. A good plan should always include cleansing, moisturizing, and protecting your skin from the sun. Hydration—both from water and the products you use—is key. Begin by washing your face morning and night with a gentle cleanser that can lift away makeup, dirt, and other buildup without causing dryness or irritation. During the day, use a moisturizer that also offers sun protection. A lightweight formula that sinks in quickly without feeling heavy works well for both the face and neck, helping to keep your skin soft and protected at the same time. At night, switch to a product that can provide deeper moisture and help support skin while you sleep—look for one with ingredients that can fight off free radicals. Don't forget your eyes either; applying an eye cream in the morning and before bed can help reduce dryness, soften the appearance of lines, and brighten the area over time.

Using sun protection early and consistently makes a big difference in the way your skin looks years from now. SPF helps prevent dryness and sun spots while keeping your skin smoother overall. If you're looking to go a step further, you can add a retinol-based product into your evening routine. Retinol helps improve skin texture and tone by encouraging the skin to renew itself more regularly. Just be sure to avoid the eye area when applying it and stick with a proper eye cream in that spot instead.

Anti-aging Products in my Twenties (20s)

It's important to realize that changes in your skin don't just show up overnight—they build gradually over time. What you see on the surface later in life is often the result of choices made years earlier. Wrinkles, uneven tone, and spots are harder to manage once they appear, so it makes more sense to take care of your skin early on. Whether you're using a simple routine or adding products that support your skin as you age, being consistent now can make a big difference in how your skin looks and feels down the line.

Components of Skincare Product in your 20s

Research has confirmed the usefulness of several key ingredients commonly found in skincare products. Sunscreens with broad-spectrum protection help reduce the appearance of dark spots, uneven tone, and discoloration caused by sun exposure. Retinol, a form of vitamin A, is known to support skin's firmness and smoothness while also helping reduce visible lines and uneven tone. Vitamin C, also known as ascorbic acid, is rich in antioxidants and supports the skin's natural repair process and collagen building, making it a valuable part of any routine aimed at keeping the skin looking clear and refreshed.

Skincare routine for different skin types in your 20s

The way your skin behaves in your twenties can depend on its type, but all skin goes through some common changes. Dry skin, for example, tends to feel smoother because of its finer texture and smaller pores, but it also shows early signs of aging more clearly, such as fine lines. This makes it important to keep the skin properly moisturized throughout the day. If your skin is oily, breakouts might still be a regular concern even after the teen years. Products that help control shine and keep excess oil in check can make a big difference. Regardless of skin type, the natural support structure of your skin—

made up of elements like collagen and elastin—starts to weaken in your twenties. This can be due to everyday exposure to free radicals that gradually break down skin cells. As a result, taking steps to care for your skin early can help manage these changes across all skin types.

Exfoliating during your twenties is one of the best habits you can develop to keep your skin looking smooth and clear. When dead skin cells collect unevenly, your complexion can look dull and feel rough, and blocked pores become more likely, leading to breakouts. Regular exfoliation helps clear out those pores and refresh your skin's surface. Using ingredients like retinol is one approach, as it helps speed up skin turnover and keeps your complexion looking even. That said, it's important not to overdo it. Using too many exfoliating products, especially mixing physical scrubs and strong acids, can dry out your skin and cause redness or irritation. Being gentle and consistent gives better results than using harsh treatments too often.

Preventative Care

Taking care of your skin in your twenties is mostly about staying ahead of potential problems. This is the time to start using sunscreen regularly, include ingredients that support skin health like vitamin C, stick to a reliable cleansing routine, and keep the skin well hydrated with ingredients like hyaluronic acid. The choices you make now form the basis for how your skin will look and feel in the years ahead. It's a simple truth: preventing damage is easier than trying to fix it once it's already there. Healthy skin responds best when it's supported every day, not just when concerns arise. The goal here is to give your skin the care it needs to stay strong, even before signs of aging show up. That means defending it against things like sun exposure, air pollution, and other daily challenges. The habits you form early tend to show up later—either as healthy skin or as skin that's been worn down by years of neglect. Focusing on protection today means you're less likely to face serious concerns down the road.

At-home care plays a major role in this. A good skincare routine should include a gentle cleanser to remove buildup and makeup, a quality moisturizer to keep the skin soft and hydrated, and daily sunscreen to protect against UV rays, even on cloudy days. Adding products that contain ingredients like vitamin C can help shield the skin from everyday stress. Retinoids are another option to consider, especially for helping skin refresh itself and for minimizing the chance of early lines forming. These steps don't have to be complicated to be effective.

If you choose to take it further, some people include cosmetic treatments in their plans as well. Procedures like microneedling, chemical peels, or laser-based therapies can support the skin's strength and surface when used correctly. Botox is sometimes used preventatively too, not just for smoothing existing lines but for keeping them from forming in the first place. When these treatments are paired with a regular at-home routine, they can help maintain a fresh and even skin tone for years to come. The idea isn't to chase perfection, but to give your skin the support it needs to stay clear, smooth, and steady as time passes.

Managing Acne in your 20s

Hormonal acne often appears in adulthood and can show up as blackheads, whiteheads, painful cysts, or inflamed bumps. It usually results from increased sebum production—an oily substance created by the skin's glands—that clogs pores and leads to breakouts. While it may not always be possible to prevent this type of acne completely, it can be controlled with proper care and treatment to reduce the chances of it recurring. This kind of acne is sometimes called adult acne and can affect anyone between the ages of 20 and 50. It doesn't only appear on the face—it can also develop on the chest, shoulders, or back. These breakouts can take different forms such as small bumps, visible blackheads or whiteheads, or deeper cystic spots. The underlying cause is usually linked to how the oil glands react to hormone fluctuations, leading to an overproduction of sebum.

In the United States, acne remains the most widespread skin concern. About 80% of people will deal with it at some point in their lives. Among adult women, around half in their twenties and about a quarter in their forties still experience acne that's tied to hormone activity. Treating this kind of acne depends on how mild or severe the breakouts are. For blackheads and whiteheads, topical creams like tretinoin are often used. Inflammatory breakouts may require a combination of topical antibiotics, retinoids, or benzoyl peroxide. For more persistent or widespread cases, oral antibiotics or medications like isotretinoin might be recommended. Deeper, painful cysts can be addressed through steroid injections, which reduce swelling and speed up healing.

There are other options as well, including simple habits like washing the face regularly with a gentle cleanser. Some people find that oral contraceptives help regulate hormones and improve skin condition. Changes to one's eating habits may also reduce flare-ups for certain individuals. Light or laser-based treatments are another route to consider for those who prefer non-medicated approaches or want to add to their current routine. While adult acne can be frustrating, it doesn't have to take over. With the right care, the skin can stay balanced, and breakouts can become less frequent and less severe.

Effective Skincare Routine for Hormonal Acne

Start by cleansing your skin twice a day with a gentle face wash that effectively removes dirt and oil without causing dryness. Choosing a cleanser with ingredients like salicylic acid or benzoyl peroxide can help clear blocked pores and reduce redness linked to hormonal acne. These ingredients support clean skin without being too aggressive, especially when used regularly. Adding the right treatments can also help. In the morning, reach for a serum or spot solution with ingredients such as niacinamide or azelaic acid. These are gentle and can help manage uneven tone or inflammation. In the evening, consider using a product that includes retinol or alpha hydroxy acids, but only a few times a week. These ingredients help with skin renewal but may be too harsh if applied too often.

Even when skin feels oily, keeping it moisturized is still important. Moisturizers that are lightweight or labeled as oil-free can help maintain balance, keeping the skin from producing even more oil in response to dryness. This is especially helpful for those dealing with hormonal breakouts. Daily sun protection is also key. Applying sunscreen every morning protects the skin from further marks and irritation that can be caused by UV rays. This step can help reduce the chance of long-term scarring or dark spots.

While a good routine at home makes a difference, professional care can offer more support. Seeing an expert for treatments like gentle extractions may help with deep blockages without creating more irritation or long-term marks. Diet can also make a noticeable difference. Choosing meals that are full of fresh fruits, vegetables, healthy fats, and whole grains can support overall balance. Reducing processed food and dairy may also help some people notice fewer breakouts. Managing daily stress can go a long way, too. Simple habits like quiet breathing exercises, stretching, or getting outside can help with overall calm.

Adding supplements may also help your skin. Most people turn to vitamin A and zinc to support clear skin. These can be included through food or with the advice of a healthcare provider. If breakouts become stubborn or painful, visiting a dermatologist is a smart step. They can offer options that are more targeted and safe to use under professional care.

Lifestyle choices also play a role. Getting enough rest each night, staying active, and supporting a healthy gut all contribute to how the skin functions. Reducing sugar, eating enough fiber and healthy fats, and avoiding habits like smoking can all help keep skin and hormones balanced over time.

Chapter Ten

Skincare in Your 30s

As we grow older, it's expected that the body will change, but sometimes these changes come sooner than they should. When signs of aging appear earlier than usual, this is often due to daily habits or exposure to outside elements. Dry skin, uneven tone, fine lines, loose texture, and spots on the skin are often among the first things people notice. While time naturally brings changes to the skin, some patterns and lifestyle choices can speed that up. Early signs may also include hair thinning, graying, or a face that begins to look less full than before.

One of the leading causes of this early aging process is the sun. The skin's exposure to strong sunlight over time weakens its structure. But sun damage is not the only issue. Other choices made daily can also wear on the skin. Thankfully, there are ways to help slow this down. Protecting your skin from the sun should become part of your everyday routine, not just something you do on vacation. Whether you're outdoors for long periods or simply heading out for errands, applying sunscreen to uncovered skin is important. A good option is a product that offers protection from both UVA and UVB rays and has an SPF of at least 30. Wearing long sleeves, wide-brimmed hats, UV-blocking sunglasses, and seeking shade also adds another layer of safety. Some clothing even comes labeled with extra UV protection.

Instead of getting a tan the traditional way, you might consider using products that give your skin a bronzed glow without sun exposure. Tanning beds and direct sun not only deepen color but also damage skin cells over time, which leads to a loss of firmness and early wrinkles. Quitting smoking is one of the best steps you can take. This habit breaks down the skin's surface and makes it appear dull and uneven. Over time, it also leads to deep lines and a loss of smoothness. Similarly, making the same facial movements over and over—like frowning or squinting—can also lead to fine lines becoming deeper and harder to treat. Wearing sunglasses helps to avoid constant squinting and the wrinkles it can bring.

Eating habits also affect your skin. Meals filled with fresh fruits and vegetables can support the skin from within. Foods with high sugar or refined ingredients, however, may add to the speed at which signs of aging appear. Cutting back on alcohol can also help. Alcohol pulls moisture out of the skin and weakens its natural ability to recover. With continued use, it can make the skin appear tired or uneven. Staying active is another step worth taking. Moving your body throughout the week improves how blood moves through the body, which can give your skin a brighter and more refreshed look.

Daily care makes a difference, too. Wash your face with a gentle cleanser rather than scrubbing. Harsh treatment can lead to irritation and long-term wear. Try to wash twice a day, especially after sweating, to keep your skin clean and fresh. Sweat that lingers—especially under hats or gear—can lead to blocked pores or breakouts.

Using a moisturizer each day helps your skin hold onto the water it needs to stay smooth and soft. If any product causes a stinging or burning feeling, that's often a sign of irritation. Products that are too strong for your skin can do more harm than good over time. Keeping your routine simple, gentle, and consistent in your thirties can go a long way in helping your skin stay healthy and feel its best.

Maintaining a Healthy Glow

To keep your skin glowing and fresh, build a steady routine that includes cleansing, exfoliating, and moisturizing. Drinking enough water throughout the day, eating meals rich in fruits and vegetables, wearing sunscreen daily, getting proper sleep, keeping stress in check, and staying active can all support your skin's appearance.

What people call "glowing skin" differs from person to person. For some, it's about skin that looks smooth and healthy—not dry, patchy, or uneven. For others, it's a soft brightness that comes naturally.

Skincare Routine

Cleanse

Wash your face every day with a gentle product that removes buildup from sweat, dirt, and the environment.

Exfoliate

Clear away dead skin regularly to keep your face looking smooth and fresh.

Moisturize

Use a product that suits your skin to hold in moisture and prevent dryness.

Sunscreen

Apply sun protection every day, no matter the weather, to help avoid long-term damage.

Avoid too much sun

While a short time in the sun can help your body, staying out for long hours can cause burns and increase the chances of long-term harm. Too much exposure can also lead to dark spots, fine lines, and other changes tied to age.

Resist from touching your face

Your hands carry oil and dirt, even after washing. Touching your face often can push that dirt into your skin, leading to blocked pores and breakouts. If you feel itchy, try using your sleeve or the back of your hand instead.

Lifestyle Habits

Drink lots of water

Hydration helps keep your skin soft and smooth. It may also help slow signs of aging like lines and sagging by keeping skin firm.

Exercise regularly

Movement helps your blood flow better, which means more oxygen and nutrients reach your skin. This supports a healthy color and helps the body flush out waste.

Get Quality Sleep

Rest gives your skin time to rebuild. While you sleep, your skin replaces old cells with new ones and produces collagen, which helps your face look full and smooth. With better collagen, there's less sagging and fewer lines.

Utilize a silk-like pillowcase

Some pillow fabrics, like cotton, soak up your skin's natural oils. This can leave your skin dry and collect oils and dead cells on the fabric, possibly leading to breakouts. Using a smoother pillowcase can be gentler on your face.

Manage stress

When you're stressed, your body makes more cortisol, a hormone that causes oil buildup, which can lead to clogged pores and acne. Stress can also trigger irritation inside the body, which may affect your skin.

Studies have connected high stress with skin issues like eczema and psoriasis.

Shower with warm water

A steamy bath might feel great, but very hot water can dry out your skin. It strips away moisture, leaving it rough and flaky. A warm shower is better, followed by a good moisturizer.

Drink less alcohol

Alcohol pulls water from your body, which can make your skin dry and dull. It can also highlight lines and bring out tired tones. Drinking often may also limit your body's supply of vitamins—like folic acid—which your skin needs to hold in moisture.

Laugh a little longer

Smiling and laughter can naturally bring color to your cheeks. That's because happy moments improve circulation in the skin. So find time for joy, hobbies, or moments that make you feel at peace.

Healthy Diet

Eat a nutritious diet

Balanced meals play a big role in how your skin looks. Make sure your plate includes fresh produce, whole grains, and lean protein. Some fruits and vegetables may help slow early signs of aging. Try to cut back on soda, sweet snacks, and heavily processed foods. These can affect skin health and have been linked to quicker aging. While it's not clear-cut, some studies link frequent milk intake and high-sugar foods to acne. Others suggest that fiber and omega-3 fats might help reduce it, but more studies are still needed.

Eat More Fruits and Vegetables

These foods are packed with nutrients and can help protect your skin. Many of them also carry water, which keeps your skin from drying out. Good options include grapes, watermelon, and celery. Try switching out packaged snacks for fruits and veggies throughout your day. Carrot sticks, berries, or cucumbers make great choices. Including them in every meal can really make a difference over time.

Increase your fiber intake

Fiber helps clean out your system, which can show up on your skin. It supports blood flow, which allows nutrients to get to your skin cells faster.

Chapter Eleven

Skincare in Your 40s and Beyond

As we move through the different stages of life, our skin begins to reflect those changes—telling its own story of time and experience. One of the more obvious signs of aging is the gradual change in how firm and tight the skin feels. This shift can show up as drooping, looseness, or a general loss of that youthful bounce. In this part, we'll take a closer look at what leads to this change, where it's most noticeable, and what can be done to help the skin look and feel more refreshed.

Skin's ability to stay firm depends on how well it can stretch and return to its usual shape after movement or shifts in body position. This ability comes from two important proteins: collagen and elastin. These are found in the deeper layer of the skin and work together to give structure and flexibility. Over time, the body starts to produce less of these proteins. When that happens, the skin becomes less firm, leading to the changes noticeable with age.

Primary causes of loss of elasticity

The natural aging process is one of the main reasons the skin begins to lose its firmness over time. As we grow older, the skin produces less collagen and elastin, which are the building blocks that help it stay smooth and tight. This gradual drop in production leads to thinner, weaker skin that doesn't hold its shape as well as it once did.

Another common reason for this change is extended time under the sun. Ultraviolet rays can break down the fibers in the skin responsible for keeping it strong and flexible. After years of exposure, these rays can cause visible changes like drooping, lines, and an overall loss of bounce—often earlier than expected. Daily habits can also play a part.

Choices like smoking, eating poorly, drinking too much alcohol, or not staying hydrated can weaken the skin over time. These habits reduce the nutrients the body needs to keep the skin looking full and smooth.

Some of these changes can come down to what runs in the family. The way our skin ages and how firm it remains may be partly shaped by our genes. In some cases, there may also be inherited skin conditions or irregularities that affect how much collagen the body makes or how the skin holds its structure.

Areas susceptible to sagging

Loss of elasticity can affect many parts of the body, though some areas tend to show it more clearly than others. It's often first noticed in the face, especially around the cheeks, along the jawline, and around the neck where the skin may start to loosen or hang slightly. Under the eyes, the skin can appear thinner or less firm, making puffiness or sagging more noticeable. The upper arms and elbows may also begin to look less toned, with the skin becoming softer and less tight over time. Around the midsection, including the stomach and waist, changes in skin tightness can also become more apparent, particularly after weight changes or pregnancy. The same goes for the thighs and buttocks, where the skin may gradually lose its former shape and support.

Techniques for restoring firmness

Topical products can be a helpful part of your daily routine when aiming to improve skin firmness. Items that include ingredients like vitamin C, peptides, retinoids, and hyaluronic acid are often used to support the skin's structure. These ingredients may help encourage the skin to produce more collagen, improve its surface, and support a firmer feel over time.

There are also treatments that don't involve surgery but still aim to improve how the skin looks and feels. Options like laser sessions, ultrasound-based methods, radio waves, or microcurrent facials are often used to firm areas that have started to loosen. These approaches work by warming the deeper parts of the skin or sending energy beneath the surface, which can trigger the body's repair process and help rebuild support from within. Making everyday choices that benefit your skin is also important. Eating well, staying active, drinking enough water, and getting good sleep all help the skin do its job better. Cutting back on smoking and limiting alcohol can also prevent further wear on your skin's appearance.

Protecting your skin from the sun is one of the best ways to avoid faster aging. Daily sunscreen is key—use one that covers both UVA and UVB rays and has an SPF of 30 or higher. When outside for long periods, reapply it at least every two hours, and try to find shade when possible. While changes in skin strength are a normal part of getting older, there are ways to manage how quickly these changes appear. By being consistent with care and making smart choices, it's possible to keep the skin looking refreshed and strong. Taking steps to care for your skin can help you move through the years feeling confident and at ease with the natural changes that come along the way.

Managing Age Spots and Wrinkles

As we grow older, small patches of discoloration can start to appear on the skin. These spots—often brown, black, or grey—tend to show up in areas that see the most sunlight, such as the shoulders, face, and hands. People may begin to notice them in their thirties or forties, especially if they've had years of sun exposure. Even if sunscreen has been a part of your routine, spending a lot of time in the sun over the years can still lead to dark marks. While those with deeper skin tones are less likely to get age spots, they may experience uneven patches of skin color in other ways. The good news is there are ways to reduce the appearance of these marks.

The best way to manage age spots is to stop them before they begin. Cutting down on time spent under direct sunlight is one of the most effective ways to protect the skin from early signs of aging. The more you protect your skin from UV rays, the less likely it is for new spots to form or existing ones to become more noticeable. If you already have age spots, there are methods to help them fade. Some people choose to try home care first. With patience, these options can lead to a visible difference after a few months. Others may decide to visit a dermatologist for treatments that are done in a clinic. Two popular choices are chemical peels and laser sessions.

Laser procedures focus directly on dark spots by targeting the pigmented areas. This treatment often requires more than one visit and is more aggressive than home remedies. However, it's not suitable for everyone. People with very dark skin tones or certain skin concerns should approach laser options carefully. It's also important to avoid this method if you're pregnant, prone to scarring, or have had cold sores near the area being treated, unless proper precautions are taken. Chemical peels are another option carried out by a professional. These involve applying a solution that contains acids like glycolic, lactic, or alpha-hydroxy. The treatment removes the upper layer of the skin, which can help reduce the look of dark spots over time.

At home, you can support your skin by using products such as exfoliators, vitamin C serums, or skin-brightening treatments. If needed, a doctor can also recommend prescription creams to assist with fading darker patches. A full guide to dealing with wrinkles was explained in Chapter 2.

Advanced treatments are also available to reduce age spots and improve the overall condition of the skin. When dealing with dark spots, there are several options that can help fade or remove them. Photo-rejuvenation uses light-based technology to target areas of uneven tone. Cryotherapy involves freezing the affected spots, causing them to lighten or fall away over time. Some people may be prescribed skin creams that contain bleaching agents such as hydroquinone, which works gradually to reduce discoloration. Microdermabrasion gently removes the surface layer of skin, helping to even out tone, while intense pulsed light uses bursts of light to target unwanted pigmentation.

For general skin concerns beyond age spots and wrinkles, a wide range of treatments can help improve appearance and texture. Chemical peels remove the top layer of skin to reveal a smoother surface. Laser sessions can target various skin issues, from dullness to uneven texture. Microdermabrasion, already mentioned for spots, can also be used more broadly for a fresher look. Collagen induction therapy, often done with fine needles, can help the skin renew itself. Injectable fillers can restore volume and smooth out fine lines. Low-level laser methods are used to support skin repair at a gentler level. Sometimes, a mix of treatments may be suggested for better results. And no matter the approach, keeping the skin moisturized remains an important part of any care routine.

Chapter Twelve

Advanced Skincare

Advanced skincare includes a wide variety of treatments performed by trained medical professionals to improve the look, function, and overall condition of the skin. Dermatologists associated with the American Society for Dermatologic Surgery (ASDS) offer both medical and cosmetic options tailored to different needs across all age groups. One such method is ambulatory phlebectomy, a technique done in a clinic setting to remove visible veins through tiny openings in the skin. Blepharoplasty is used to lift drooping eyelids by taking out loose skin and fat from around the eyes. Cellfina is another option used in one session to smooth out dimples caused by cellulite, especially on the thighs and buttocks.

Chemical peels involve applying a solution that removes the outer skin layer, revealing a smoother surface underneath. These are used for uneven tone, acne scars, dark spots, sagging skin, and other signs of aging. Cryolipolysis, often called fat freezing or by its brand name CoolSculpting, works by applying controlled cooling to break down fat without harming the surrounding skin. Cryosurgery uses freezing temperatures to remove spots, unwanted growths, or early skin cancer. Dermabrasion uses a rotating tool to smooth the top layer of the skin, helping improve scars, wrinkles, and discoloration. Dermal fillers temporarily restore volume to areas like the lips or cheeks and can soften facial lines and marks.

Hair transplant procedures involve moving hair from one part of the scalp to areas where hair is thinning. Injectable calcium hydroxylapatite (CaHA), known under the brand name Radiesse, is used to reduce the appearance of deep folds in the face and correct volume loss from certain health conditions. Deoxycholic acid, sold as Kybella, is used to reduce fullness under the chin without surgery. Hyaluronic acid fillers draw in water and give the skin a plumper look. These are often used to refresh areas of the face that have lost their bounce. Poly-L-lactic acid, marketed as Sculptra, is approved to treat facial fat loss, especially in patients with HIV. Another option is polymethylmethacrylate (PMMA), sold as Bellafill, which combines microspheres with collagen and is used to improve deep facial lines.

Laser and light-based procedures treat several skin concerns such as dark spots, fine lines, unwanted hair, and visible blood vessels. Laser resurfacing removes outer skin layers to smooth texture and lessen the appearance of scars, wrinkles, and sagging areas. Liposuction is a surgical method to remove fat from specific parts of the body through suction. Microdermabrasion uses a device with a mildly abrasive tip to remove the skin's outer layer and refresh its surface. Micro-lipoinjection transfers fat from one area of the body to another to fill in wrinkles or restore fullness. Microneedling uses fine needles to make small channels in the skin, which may help improve texture and tone.

Micropigmentation, also called permanent makeup, is used to restore color to the skin, including in cases of scarring or pigment loss. Microwave thermolysis is a treatment for controlling excessive sweating. A neck lift is a surgical procedure used to improve the appearance of the neck and usually offers long-lasting changes. Neuromodulators, such as botulinum toxin injections, reduce the look of lines by relaxing facial muscles. These are used for forehead lines, crow's feet, and other expressions that cause creasing. Non-ablative laser methods use heat to trigger skin repair without removing layers of skin, helping with wrinkles and blemishes.

There are also several ways to shape the body without surgery. Some use gentle lasers, ultrasound, or radio waves to reduce fat. Treatments that tighten the skin without surgery often rely on devices that work beneath the surface to slowly improve firmness by encouraging the skin to rebuild its structure over time.

Chemical Peels

Chemical peels involve a step-by-step process where the skin is first cleaned and stripped of surface oils. After that, a chemical solution is applied to the area being treated. This causes the skin to blister and gradually peel off, revealing a layer of newer skin underneath that tends to look fresher and smoother. This procedure is commonly used to help reduce the appearance of wrinkles, uneven skin tone, scars, age spots, freckles, dark patches like melasma, and certain forms of acne. It works by removing damaged skin layers to allow healthier skin to surface. The kind of chemical peel you receive depends on the skin issue you're aiming to treat. There are three general levels.

A light peel, also known as a superficial peel, targets the outermost layer of the skin. It can help with fine lines, dryness, acne, and mild discoloration. This type can be done more than once, often spaced a few weeks apart, depending on how your skin reacts. A medium peel removes cells from both the surface and part of the middle layer of the skin. It's commonly chosen for deeper wrinkles, acne marks, or uneven skin tone. In some cases, more than one session may be needed for better results. A deep peel goes further into the skin to treat more pronounced wrinkles, scars, or skin growths that may need medical attention. This option is more intense and usually delivers lasting results after a single treatment, meaning no follow-up sessions are needed unless advised otherwise. Chemical peels may also be referred to as chemexfoliation or derma-peeling, depending on the context or the technique used.

Microdermabrasion

Microdermabrasion begins with cleansing the skin using a gentle product to remove surface oils and dirt. The eyes are then covered to protect them during the procedure. A device, either using a stream of tiny crystals or a wand with a diamond tip, is used to glide across the skin. As the skin is gently abraded, a suction tool removes the loosened particles and dead cells. Any remaining debris is wiped away with a soft cloth, and a moisturizer is applied to soothe the skin.

There are two main approaches to this treatment. Crystal microdermabrasion involves spraying fine crystals onto the skin, which helps exfoliate the outer layer. In diamond microdermabrasion, a hand-held tool with a diamond tip is used instead, offering a more controlled and precise way to remove dull skin. People often choose this method to smooth out rough patches, reduce uneven skin tone, and address concerns like melasma, sun-related changes, mild scarring, or stretch marks. It can also help fade dark spots, unclog pores, and improve how the skin absorbs moisturizing products. As circulation improves during the process, the skin may appear brighter and more refreshed. This treatment suits a wide range of skin types and generally comes with minimal side effects. Afterward, the skin might look pink or feel slightly sensitive, but this usually fades within a few days.

Laser Treatments

Laser treatments are carried out through a process that begins with the specialist directing a focused beam of light onto a specific area of the body. A precise device is used to concentrate the light on the chosen spot. Once the light is applied, the tissue absorbs the energy, leading to effects such as heating, destruction of certain cells, or sealing of vessels—depending on the laser's wavelength and purpose. The skin responds to this energy by triggering a repair process, which can lead to visible results like smoother texture, tighter skin, or removal of unwanted growths.

There are several types of laser and light-based treatments, each developed to target particular skin concerns. Some are designed for deep resurfacing, while others are more gentle and focus on overall improvement with shorter recovery periods. Ablative lasers, such as CO_2 and Erbium YAG, remove outer layers of the skin by vaporizing tissue. These lasers rely on water in the skin to absorb the light energy, which then breaks down damaged areas on the surface and below. This method is often used for more advanced concerns like deep wrinkles, large scars, or lesions. Because the process involves removing both surface and deeper layers, healing time tends to be longer.

Non-ablative lasers, such as Nd and Diode lasers, treat the underlying layers without removing the outer skin. These work by gently heating the tissue beneath the surface, which can encourage firmness and smoother texture over time. This approach is often used for more moderate concerns, like minor lines, dark spots, or visible veins. Since the top layer remains intact, recovery is usually quicker, though results appear more gradually.

Fractional lasers, including fractional CO_2 and fractional Erbium, combine the approaches of both ablative and non-ablative lasers. These devices treat small sections of the skin at a time by creating controlled, tiny wounds surrounded by untouched tissue. This method allows the skin to recover faster while still encouraging collagen production and improving skin tone and texture. Fractional lasers are often chosen for wrinkle smoothing, resurfacing, and scar reduction, as they strike a balance between effectiveness and recovery time.

Pulsed dye lasers work by aiming light at the blood vessels in the skin, particularly focusing on the red pigment found in the blood. These are commonly used for skin concerns such as redness, spider veins, or conditions like rosacea. The light is absorbed by the blood, causing the targeted vessel to shrink or close without harming nearby areas.

Q-switched lasers deliver light in powerful bursts that last for a very short time. These lasers are well-suited for removing tattoos and treating dark patches. They work by breaking up pigment particles using a quick energy pulse, which allows the body to clear away the pigment naturally. This method is precise, helping to reduce unwanted color without causing widespread damage to the surrounding skin.

Laser treatments are used in a wide range of areas. In skincare, they help with smoothing out wrinkles, treating scars, fading dark spots, and managing redness from visible veins. For hair removal, lasers aim at melanin in the hair to damage the follicle and reduce future growth. In medical care, they are used in eye surgeries like LASIK to improve vision or treat pressure in glaucoma. Lasers also assist in targeting cancer cells in specific body regions and removing unwanted blood vessels such as spider veins. Each use is based on the laser's ability to deliver focused energy to precise areas, allowing for controlled treatment and targeted results.

Botox and Fillers

Botox and fillers are common treatments used to smooth out wrinkles and restore volume in areas that have started to lose firmness with time. In the case of Botox, a very small dose of botulinum toxin is carefully injected into the specific muscle responsible for causing a wrinkle. This substance works by relaxing that muscle, preventing it from contracting, which softens the appearance of lines that usually form when making facial expressions. It doesn't affect the entire face, just the targeted area, allowing surrounding muscles to continue moving normally.

Fillers, on the other hand, involve injecting a gel-like material just beneath the skin. These substances are usually made from hyaluronic acid, collagen, or calcium hydroxylapatite. The purpose is to fill in lines, folds, or places where the skin has thinned or sagged, which gives the face a more full and youthful shape. Fillers don't interfere with muscle movement but instead focus on adding volume or structure where it's been lost.

Though Botox is widely recognized by name, it is actually a specific brand. Similar products include Xeomin, Jeuveau, and Dysport, all of which serve the same function but may vary slightly in how they are formulated. When it comes to fillers, there are several types as well. Hyaluronic acid fillers are among the most used and include options like Belotero, Restylane, and Juvederm. These come in various consistencies to suit different areas of the face. Collagen-based fillers are generally selected for fine lines, while calcium hydroxylapatite options are more often used for deeper folds or areas that need added structure, like the cheeks. Poly-L-lactic acid, sold under the name Sculptra, is known for stimulating the skin's own collagen production over time, offering gradual improvement in facial volume.

The main difference between these treatments lies in how they work. Botox targets the muscle underneath the skin, which helps to reduce the movement that leads to expression lines. This makes it a good option for areas like frown lines, lines across the forehead, and the fine creases around the eyes. Fillers, by contrast, are more often used to address areas where the skin has lost thickness or shape. Common uses include plumping the lips, softening the lines from the nose to the mouth, filling hollows under the eyes, or lifting the cheeks for a more rounded contour. Each approach serves its own purpose, and they are often used together to achieve a more balanced and refreshed appearance.

Chapter Thirteen

DIY Treatments at Home

At-home peels are skincare treatments you can apply yourself using exfoliating powders or liquid solutions. These formulas contain acids or enzymes that, once applied, begin to work through the outer layer of the skin. By loosening the bonds that keep dead skin cells attached, the solution helps clear the surface and makes way for new, smoother skin to appear. This process helps refresh your complexion, leaving it looking brighter and more even.

The way these peels work is by softening the material that holds older skin cells in place. As those cells are lifted away, your skin responds by speeding up its natural repair cycle. This includes increased production of collagen, which over time can lead to firmer and more resilient skin. One reason most persons turn to these treatments is that they offer a more affordable and convenient option compared to in-office sessions. With the ability to adjust both the ingredients and their strength, you can tailor each peel to suit your own skin type and sensitivity. This gives you the flexibility to address specific issues, like dullness, rough patches, or early signs of aging, without leaving your home.

Types of Do-it-yourself Chemical Peels

When it comes to at-home chemical peels, there are many options to choose from, each offering its own approach and effects. Among the most common types used in homemade skincare routines are alpha-hydroxy acids, or AHAs. Glycolic acid, which is sourced from sugar cane, is often chosen for its ability to reach beneath the surface and support the natural renewal of skin cells. It's a go-to for those who want to improve texture and reduce the appearance of fine lines. Lactic acid, derived from milk, works in a much gentler way. It not only exfoliates but also helps the skin stay hydrated, which makes it a good fit for people with sensitivity. There are also fruit-based acids like citric from citrus fruits, malic from apples, and tartaric from grapes. These provide light exfoliation and are well-suited to those trying peels for the first time or dealing with delicate skin.

Beta hydroxy acids are another group, with salicylic acid being the most widely used. Since it's oil-soluble, it works well for oily or acne-prone skin, clearing out pores and reducing irritation. In addition to acids, enzymes from fruits like papaya and pineapple are used to gently loosen dead skin without causing too much stress to the surface. Papain and bromelain are especially helpful for people looking for a mild yet effective option. With a better sense of what each ingredient can offer, it's possible to create basic peels at home using a few simple items. A glycolic acid peel can be made by mixing one tablespoon of glycolic acid at a 30% concentration with one tablespoon of purified water. This is applied to clean skin and left on for just two to three minutes before rinsing. For a lactic acid peel, plain yogurt can be combined with honey—two tablespoons of yogurt with one teaspoon of honey—and applied to the skin for ten to fifteen minutes before washing it off. A salicylic acid peel can be prepared by mixing one teaspoon of a 2% solution with a tablespoon of aloe vera gel, applying it for five to ten minutes, and then rinsing thoroughly. A fruit-based option like a papaya peel can be created by mashing a quarter cup of ripe papaya and combining it with one tablespoon of honey. This blend can stay on the skin for ten to fifteen minutes before removal.

Before trying any of these peels, it's important to prepare your skin properly and gather the items you'll need. The first step is to perform a patch test. Apply a small amount of the peel to a discreet area, such as behind the ear, and wait 24 hours to check for any reaction. If the skin stays calm, you can move forward. Start by cleansing your face thoroughly to remove dirt, oil, or any makeup. Avoid other exfoliating treatments for at least a day beforehand to lower the chance of irritation. Make sure you have your ingredients measured, a bowl and spoon for mixing, cotton pads or a small brush for applying, and a neutralizing mix like baking soda with water ready in case you need to calm the skin afterward.

Once everything is set, apply the peel evenly over clean, dry skin using your tool of choice. If it's your first time, test how your skin responds by using a thin layer and adjusting in future uses based on comfort. Leave the mixture on for the time suggested based on the ingredient and how your skin handles it. Rinse thoroughly with lukewarm water, or use your neutralizer if necessary. Some general precautions are important to keep in mind. Never use a peel on broken or irritated skin. Be careful to avoid the eyes and the area around them, and don't apply near the mouth or nose openings. If the skin starts to burn or sting more than expected, rinse immediately and stop the session. After the treatment, apply a gentle, non-pore-blocking moisturizer to calm and hydrate your skin. It's also essential to apply sunscreen with at least SPF 30, as your skin will be more exposed to sun damage for several days.

In the days that follow, stick with mild products to avoid stressing the skin. Sunscreen should continue to be a daily step, especially if you plan to keep doing peels in the future. Depending on how well your skin tolerates the process and the changes you're looking for, you can repeat the peel every two to four weeks. This regular care can support long-term skin improvement while letting your skin recover fully between treatments.

Microneedling Devices

To perform microneedling at home, you'll need a few basic items, including a roller device, 70% isopropyl alcohol, a gentle cleanser, and a serum to apply after the treatment. A numbing cream can also be used if you're sensitive to discomfort, especially when working with longer needles. Begin by disinfecting the roller. Let it soak in 70% isopropyl alcohol for about five to ten minutes. This is an important step to avoid introducing bacteria to your skin. While the roller is soaking, cleanse your face thoroughly with a mild, pH-balanced cleanser to remove any dirt or oil. Once your skin is clean, you can swipe your face with a bit of the alcohol to ensure it's fully prepped. If you find microneedling uncomfortable, applying a numbing cream after cleansing and before rolling can help. For those using longer needles, numbing becomes even more useful.

Once your skin is ready, divide your face into four sections in your mind—upper left, upper right, lower left, and lower right—while steering clear of the eye area. Pick one section to begin with and roll gently in one direction, either vertically or horizontally, two to three times. After each pass, lift the roller rather than dragging it back and forth. Once you've covered that section in one direction, shift slightly and continue until the area is done. Then repeat the process across the same section, but this time change direction so that the pattern crosses over the first. This cross-motion helps make sure the skin is evenly treated.

After you've completed all areas, rinse your face with clean water and pat it dry with a fresh cloth or cotton pad. At this point, it's time to clean your derma roller again. First, rinse it with dish soap and warm water. Then soak it in 70% isopropyl alcohol for another ten minutes. After that, allow it to dry and place it back in its container. Be sure to replace your roller after about ten to fifteen uses, or even sooner if you use it several times a week. Keeping your tools clean and in good condition is just as important as the treatment itself to keep your skin safe and the process effective.

LED Light Therapy

When it comes to skincare, creativity plays a major role in finding what truly works. Gone are the days when routines stopped at cleansers, moisturizers, toners, and serums. These remain key to healthy skin, but technology has opened the door to treatments that go beyond the basics. One of the most talked-about additions in recent years is LED light therapy. Though the use of light-emitting diodes isn't new, their application in skincare has drawn growing interest and praise in beauty circles.

LED light therapy is a gentle, non-invasive method that uses infrared light at different wavelengths to target skin concerns. These lights reach below the surface to encourage natural processes within the skin. This method didn't start in beauty clinics; it was first developed for medical use. Back in the 1990s, the U.S. Navy SEALs used LED therapy to speed up the recovery of wounds and muscle injuries. NASA also saw its potential, especially for astronauts in space, where limited gravity, oxygen, and sunlight affected healing. Without the right conditions, their cells didn't repair or multiply as they would on Earth. LED light provided the push needed to help cells renew and rebuild, which sparked further interest in its broader uses.

Since then, the focus has shifted toward its effects on skin. Each color of LED light is selected based on its ability to target a specific concern. Some are used to boost the skin's firmness by encouraging collagen and elastin, while others help with breakouts by calming inflammation and balancing oil levels. The treatment can also support healing in damaged tissues and reduce the appearance of wrinkles or dark spots. Devices that use LED therapy come with different light settings such as blue, amber, red, yellow, and green. Each color is absorbed by different receptors within the skin, sending energy into the cells and triggering various responses. What makes this method appealing is how each color reaches a different depth, creating changes based on how far into the skin it travels. To get the best results, it's important to know which light frequency suits your specific concern. Each setting has a unique purpose, and using the right one can help you reach your skincare goals more effectively. LED therapy is appropriate for all skin types and tones. Individuals who have rosacea can also use LED light face treatments.

Red LED Light Therapy

Red LED light, also known as infrared light, works by targeting the skin's surface layer, called the epidermis. It's often used to calm inflammation and ease signs of aging. The lighter shades within the red spectrum are known to help reduce visible redness and support healthy blood flow. The deeper end of the red light range reaches further into the skin, focusing on cell activity and recovery. When this light is absorbed, it signals fibroblast cells to increase their production of collagen and elastin. These two proteins are essential for giving skin its firmness and shape, which can result in a more filled-out, youthful appearance.

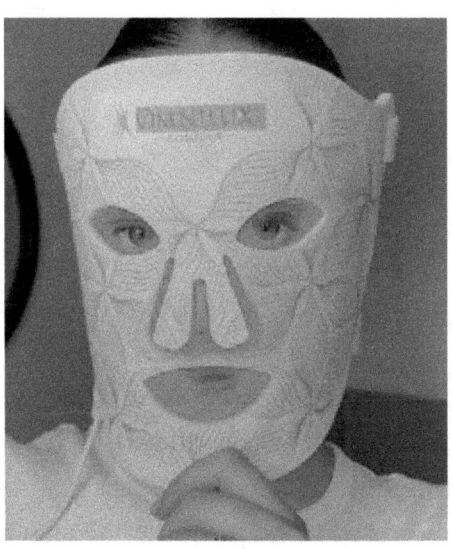

In addition to its skin-related use, some studies have also noted that red LED light may help improve hair thickness, slow down shedding, and encourage new strands to grow in people dealing with inherited hair loss. Because of its potential to support both skin and scalp health, this type of light is commonly included in LED masks designed for home use.

Blue LED light therapy

Blue LED light therapy works by focusing on the skin's oil-producing glands. This specific type of light can help reduce excess oil, clear out the pores, and play a role in calming breakouts. It's often chosen for its ability to target bacteria linked to acne without irritating the skin. The light reaches beneath the surface to disrupt the growth of these bacteria, which are known to contribute to different types of blemishes, from small whiteheads to more stubborn cystic spots and nodules. Because it doesn't involve harsh ingredients or manual scrubbing, it's often well-tolerated even by those with sensitive skin.

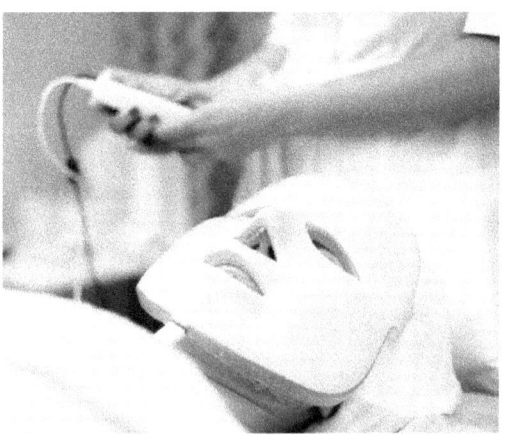

This light setting is also being used to manage skin conditions like eczema and psoriasis, offering a gentler option for relief. For even better results, pairing blue light with red light can be useful—blue to tackle the bacteria and red to help soothe the skin and reduce visible redness. Together, they offer a balanced approach to clearer, calmer skin.

Green LED Light Therapy

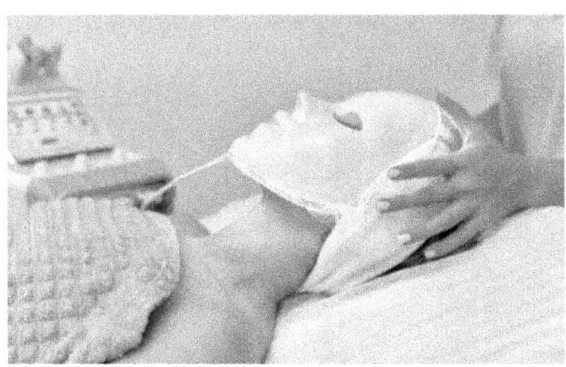

Green LED light therapy is often used to target uneven skin tone caused by issues like dark circles, discoloration, sunspots, and visible blood vessels near the surface. It works to create a more balanced look across the skin by calming areas where color may be uneven or too intense. This type of light reaches the lower part of the skin's outermost layer, where melanin-producing cells are located. Its action helps slow down the overproduction of melanin, which is the pigment responsible for darker spots. By keeping excess pigment from rising to the surface, it can help support a clearer, more even-toned appearance over time.

Yellow LED Light Therapy

Yellow LED light therapy reaches into the deeper layers of the skin, where it connects with specific receptors in the cells. It is often chosen for helping to soften the look of fine lines, creases, and other age-related changes. This light setting also plays a role in supporting better blood flow just beneath the surface, which can give the skin a healthier tone and help calm areas of redness. Regular use of yellow light treatments may support a smoother and more refreshed appearance without causing discomfort or stress to the skin.

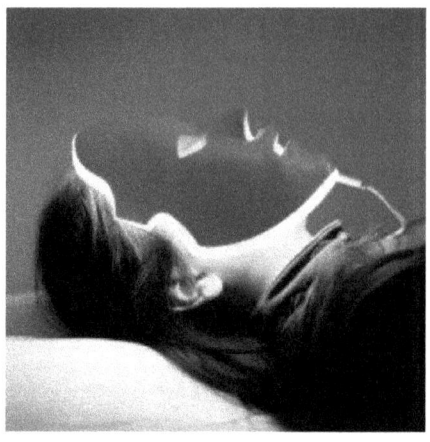

White LED Light Therapy

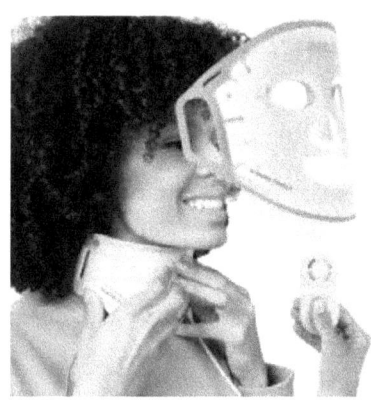

White LED light therapy, often referred to as near-infrared light, has the longest wavelength among the available LED options. Because of this, it can reach deeper layers of the skin compared to other light settings. This deeper reach supports skin from the inside out, helping it stay strong and balanced beneath the surface while improving how it looks on the outside. Most users turn to white LED light to improve the appearance of acne scars, firm up loose skin, calm redness, and reduce marks caused by sun exposure. It's a gentle but steady option for those wanting to support their skin in a way that goes beyond the surface. When going through sessions, you can choose a single light color to focus on a specific goal or combine different wavelengths for a more customized approach.

You can go for full-body LED beds to refresh your entire system or stick to facial light treatments, either through professional sessions or at-home LED face masks. In-salon options are usually offered in spas, skincare clinics, dermatologists' offices, or by licensed aestheticians. A single session often takes about 20 minutes. Since light-based skin support works gradually, you may be asked to come in for ten or more visits to get noticeable results.

If you prefer staying in, you can still enjoy the benefits without having to schedule a visit. With at-home LED light devices now widely available, it's possible to support your skin from your own bathroom or bedroom. These tools are easy to use, and you don't need any special training to start. To begin, always start by washing your face. Clean skin allows the light to reach more effectively, and removing buildup from your pores is important before applying the device. After drying your skin completely, place the LED mask or device on your face. You can start with shorter sessions—around 10 minutes—and gradually work your way up to about 30 minutes, two or three times a week, depending on how your skin reacts. To complete your routine, you might choose to apply a serum or facial oil. While this step isn't required, it can leave your skin feeling softer and looking smoother after the treatment.

When not to Use LED Light Therapy

It's important to keep in mind that certain health conditions may not pair well with LED light facial treatments. If any of the following apply to you, it's best to be cautious when considering this method or using LED face masks at home. People dealing with an active skin rash, frequent migraines, or a history of seizures should consult with a professional before starting. Those with epilepsy or existing eye problems may also need to avoid this treatment due to light sensitivity. If there is any current bleeding or if you've been diagnosed with cancer, it's best to hold off entirely unless advised otherwise by a doctor. The same goes for those who are pregnant—while the treatment may seem gentle, it's still a good idea to wait or check with a healthcare provider before moving forward.

Chapter Fourteen

Some Skincare Myths

"You Don't Need Sunscreen Indoors" is one of those widely believed myths that continues to cause confusion. People assume that sunscreen is only necessary when stepping outside or spending time in direct sunlight. Being indoors often gives a false sense of security, as if walls and windows offer complete protection. But in reality, that's far from the case. Ultraviolet A (UVA) rays can pass through glass and still reach your skin, even if you're inside. These rays are known to contribute to early signs of aging, uneven skin tone, and long-term damage that may lead to serious conditions.

There's also the added concern of blue light exposure. Devices like phones, tablets, and computer screens release this type of light, and while it may not cause an immediate burn, it can still play a role in developing fine lines, pigmentation, and other changes in skin texture over time. This is why wearing sunscreen indoors—especially a mineral-based one—is a smart habit, not just for sun-filled days, but even when you're spending hours in front of screens or sitting near windows. Cloudy skies also don't mean your skin is safe. According to the Skin Cancer Foundation, clouds only block around a quarter of ultraviolet rays. That leaves most of the harmful radiation still reaching your skin. For proper daily care, it's a good idea to apply sunscreen as the last step in your morning routine—regardless of the weather or whether you're going out or staying in.

"Pores Can Open and Close" is a claim that sounds convincing but doesn't hold up to how the skin actually works. Pores don't have muscles, so they're not capable of physically opening or closing. What often leads to this misunderstanding is the temporary change in how pores look depending on skin temperature or what products are used. For example, warm steam can soften the buildup inside pores, making it easier to clean out trapped oil and debris. This might give the impression that the pores are opening, but what's really happening is that the contents inside are loosening. On the other hand, applying something cold to the skin, like chilled water or a cool compress, may make pores appear smaller. This effect is brief and cosmetic, not a result of the pores actually shrinking. When pores are filled with excess oil or dirt, they can look larger than they really are, which makes them more noticeable. Cleaning out that buildup can help them look smoother, but again, it doesn't mean they've closed. The idea that pores can open and shut like doors has stuck around for a long time, but what you're really seeing is how they react to different conditions, not an actual change in their structure.

"Natural Oils Are Always Safe" is an idea that sounds comforting, but it doesn't always hold true. Just because something is plant-based or naturally sourced doesn't mean it will suit every skin type. Some natural oils are known to clog pores, which can lead to breakouts and irritation—especially for people with sensitive or acne-prone skin. Coconut oil is often praised for its moisturizing benefits, yet it's one of the more comedogenic oils and can worsen skin concerns for some individuals. Olive oil falls into a similar category; while it may work well for dry skin, it's not the best fit for all areas or all people.

Before adding any new oil to your routine, especially on delicate skin, it's best to do a patch test. What feels gentle and nourishing to one person might cause redness, itching, or bumps in another. Some natural oils also disrupt the skin's natural balance, leaving behind a greasy layer that traps sweat, bacteria, and other impurities. This can lead to blocked pores, unpleasant odor, or inflammation—particularly in areas that are already sensitive. There's also the issue of moisture. While oils can seal in hydration, they don't provide water-based moisture on their own. This means they may not deliver the hydration your skin actually needs, especially in intimate or easily irritated areas. If your skin is reactive or prone to dryness, skipping proper hydration can lead to dryness beneath the surface, even if the skin feels soft at first.

When it comes to acne, the idea that all natural oils are harmless is especially misleading. Oils like coconut or olive oil may feel smooth going on, but they can make clogged pores worse. On the other hand, there are options that are far less likely to cause trouble. Tea tree oil and jojoba oil, for example, are known to work better with skin that needs more balance and less buildup. Choosing the right oil comes down to knowing your skin's needs, not just trusting the label or the trend. Natural doesn't always mean risk-free.

Chapter Fifteen

Lifestyle and Skincare

Caring for your skin goes beyond the surface. While quality skincare products play a role, what you eat and how well you stay hydrated are just as important. I believe that true skin wellness starts from within, and that a balanced diet along with proper hydration can do a great deal in supporting clear, smooth, and vibrant skin. Understanding how the food you eat affects your skin helps you make better choices for long-term skin health. Your daily meals have a direct effect on how your skin looks and feels. When your diet is filled with nourishing foods, your skin tends to reflect that care. Nutrient-rich ingredients like spinach, berries, dark chocolate, and nuts are packed with antioxidants that help protect the skin from free radicals—those unstable molecules that contribute to fine lines, dryness, and uneven tone. These antioxidants are especially helpful in keeping your skin looking fresh and youthful.

Vitamins like A, C, and E also play a major role in skin repair. Foods such as carrots, sweet potatoes, almonds, and oranges supply these important nutrients. Vitamin C, in particular, supports the production of collagen, a protein that keeps the skin firm and helps slow down the appearance of lines and sagging. Healthy fats are another key part of the puzzle. Omega-3 fatty acids, which you can find in foods like salmon, flaxseeds, mackerel, and walnuts, are known to reduce surface irritation and help with conditions like acne and dry patches. They also keep the skin feeling soft and looking more even by locking in moisture. Zinc is another important mineral, found in shellfish, pumpkin seeds, and chickpeas, which helps keep oil production under control and supports healing from breakouts or other irritations.

Protein-rich foods help provide structure to the skin by supporting the formation of collagen and elastin. These proteins give the skin its firmness and bounce. Including foods like tofu, lentils, beans, and lean meats in your routine helps maintain that smooth and supported look. What you eat can either build your skin up or work against it—so focusing on wholesome, nutrient-rich options is one of the smartest steps toward lasting skin health.

The Importance of Hydration in Skin Health

Keeping your skin hydrated is just as important as choosing the right foods. Water plays a major role in maintaining moisture levels and helping your body clear out waste. When your skin is properly hydrated, it's more resilient and less prone to fine lines and dryness. Drinking enough water each day supports elasticity and gives the skin a smoother, softer appearance. Staying hydrated also helps improve circulation, which allows nutrients to reach skin cells more efficiently. This can result in a clearer tone, fewer blemishes, and a natural glow.

To keep your skin in good shape, it helps to build daily habits that support both hydration and nutrition. Eating meals that include a mix of fruits, vegetables, lean protein, and healthy fats ensures you're giving your skin what it needs to stay firm and bright. Drinking water throughout the day is key, and if plain water isn't appealing, you can add fruits like cucumber, lemon, or berries to improve the taste and add extra nutrients.

Limiting highly processed foods and sugary snacks can make a big difference too. These items are often linked to surface irritation and breakouts, while whole foods tend to support smoother, calmer skin. Alcohol and caffeinated drinks can dry out the skin, so it's a good idea to follow them up with extra water when you do have them.

Eating water-rich foods like oranges, watermelon, and cucumbers can also help increase your hydration. These can be especially helpful on hot days or when your skin feels dry. It's also important to pay attention to how your skin responds to different foods. If you notice breakouts, dryness, or other changes, adjusting your diet may help restore balance.

Getting that healthy, fresh look isn't just about what you apply on the outside. A mix of the right care products, balanced meals, and steady hydration will help your skin stay smooth and clear. If you're dealing with ongoing skin concerns or not sure which steps to take, speaking with a dermatologist can provide guidance that's suited to your skin type and goals. With consistency and the right approach, you can support your skin's health from within.

Foods for Healthy Skin

A wide variety of nutrient-rich foods in your daily meals can do wonders for your skin's appearance and condition. Fatty fish like salmon, mackerel, and herring are rich in omega-3s, which help maintain a soft and hydrated complexion. Fruits such as strawberries, watermelon, cherries, red grapes, and blood oranges are packed with antioxidants that protect the skin from daily stress. Avocados, walnuts, flax seeds, sunflower seeds, and almonds are full of healthy fats and vitamins that support the skin's barrier and keep it feeling smooth.

Vegetables like red and yellow bell peppers, broccoli, spinach, carrots, kale, sweet potatoes, yams, and papayas provide vitamins and plant compounds that brighten the skin and encourage firmness. Tomatoes and soybeans offer plant-based support for smoother skin, while green tea and dark chocolate add helpful compounds that protect against environmental stressors.

Olive oil can be a flavorful way to get more skin-supporting fats in your meals, and bone broth contributes collagen, which supports skin structure from within. Shellfish, trout, oysters, and organ meats deliver minerals like zinc and iron, both of which are needed for healing and overall skin strength. Mangoes and eggs bring together a mix of vitamins, healthy fats, and proteins that all help with repair and texture. And if you're looking for a refreshing option, smoothies made with a blend of these ingredients can provide an easy and tasty way to nourish your skin daily.

Stress and Sleep

The connection between your mind and your skin is closer than most people realize. Your skin, being the largest organ, plays a major role in protecting your body from outside threats. When stress levels rise, your brain sets off a chain reaction that triggers the body's built-in defense system, often referred to as the fight-or-flight response. This activates a group of glands that produce cortisol, a hormone involved in regulating sleep patterns, blood sugar, and blood pressure, while also helping the body manage tension. However, when cortisol levels stay high for too long, it starts to affect the skin in several ways.

One of the most common effects is the increase in oil production from the sebaceous glands. Extra oil on the skin can block pores, which may lead to breakouts and clogged areas. At the same time, cortisol binds to certain cells and speeds up the loss of elastin and collagen—two key proteins that keep the skin firm and smooth. Cortisol also communicates with mast cells, which are part of the immune system. These cells react to perceived threats, sometimes leading to flare-ups such as itching, redness, or allergic responses on the skin. The brain's reaction to pressure also releases small signaling proteins known as cytokines. These molecules are responsible for triggering inflammation. While inflammation helps defend the body, too much can break down the skin's natural barrier. That top layer plays a role in protecting against germs, UV exposure, and moisture loss. When disrupted by excess cytokines, the skin may become dry, more sensitive, and prone to irritation.

Stress doesn't only affect how your skin looks—it can influence your nails and hair too. You might notice changes in how your skin feels or heals when you're going through a demanding period. In fact, stress can delay recovery from skin problems and make them more difficult to manage. This is why some people notice more frequent breakouts or skin issues when they're under pressure. That's not by chance—it's a direct response to the body's internal state. Ongoing stress can also cause flare-ups of chronic conditions like eczema, psoriasis, and rosacea. It may even lead to hives, rashes, or cold sores returning unexpectedly. What makes things worse is that stress can also interrupt everyday skincare habits. You might skip steps in your routine, stop using certain products, or feel too tired to take care of your skin properly. And for some, the appearance of a flare-up adds another layer of worry, creating a cycle that's hard to break. If you're dealing with a skin issue that keeps coming back, it may be worth thinking about how stress fits into the picture. Adjusting how you handle those triggers could be just as helpful as the products you use.

Tips for Better Sleep and Skin Recovery

Getting enough sleep each night plays a major role in both your physical and mental well-being, but that doesn't mean it's always easy. Poor sleep affects everything—mood, energy, focus, and even how your skin looks. Your daily routines, often called sleep hygiene, can influence how well you rest. According to data pulled from over 160,000 profiles on the Sleep Foundation, most people reported ongoing trouble with sleep that lasted for months or even years. There are practical steps that can help you shift into a better rhythm. From adjusting your environment to small changes in your routine, these actions can help you fall asleep faster, stay asleep longer, and wake up feeling more refreshed.

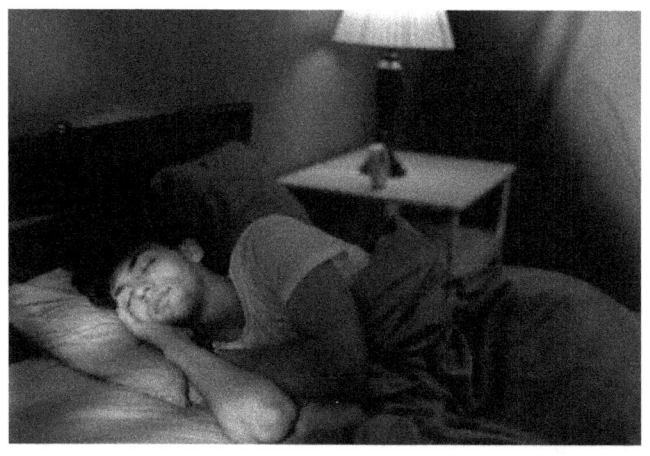

Start with where you sleep. A good mattress and pillow can make a noticeable difference. Your spine needs proper support, and your body needs a soft, temperature-friendly surface to truly relax. Bedding that feels good on your skin and maintains a steady temperature through the night can be just as important as the mattress beneath it. Lighting plays a big part too. Bright light can interfere with your body's ability to prepare for rest. Adding blackout curtains or using a sleep mask can help block out unwanted brightness. This quiet, dark setting allows your body to produce melatonin—the hormone that signals it's time to wind down. Keeping your sleep area quiet is another helpful step. If outside noise is unavoidable, try using a fan, white noise device, or earplugs to cancel it out.

Your room should also be kept at a comfortable temperature. Most people sleep best when the air is slightly cool, somewhere between 65 and 68 degrees Fahrenheit. Finding the right balance helps prevent tossing and turning due to feeling too warm or too cold. Planning enough time for rest is necessary. You need at least seven hours of sleep, so think about what time you need to wake up and count backward to choose a bedtime that gives you that full amount. Stick to a set wake-up time, even on weekends, to help your body stay on a regular rhythm.

If you take naps, try to keep them short—about twenty minutes—and aim for early in the afternoon, right after lunch. Longer or late naps can throw off your sleep later that night. Try to spend at least half an hour before bed doing something that relaxes your body and mind. Read a book, stretch gently, listen to soft music, or focus on breathing exercises to help you wind down. Rather than trying to force yourself to sleep, focus on easing into rest.

Avoid screens close to bedtime. The light from phones, tablets, and computers can keep your brain active and reduce melatonin levels, making it harder to switch off. Set a goal to stop using screens at least one hour before going to bed.

Your body's rhythm is also shaped by sunlight. Getting outside or opening the blinds for natural light during the morning can help keep your internal clock on track. If access to sunlight is limited, a light therapy box could be an option worth discussing with your doctor. Daily movement helps too. Just twenty minutes of activity each day can improve your ability to sleep. While regular workouts are good, try not to do anything intense too close to bedtime, since that can make it harder to relax.

Caffeine is a common obstacle to sleep. Drinks like coffee, tea, and soda are often used to fight daytime fatigue, but too much—especially after 2 p.m.—can keep you up at night. Alcohol also affects how you sleep. It might make you feel tired at first, but it can interfere with sleep quality and cause you to wake up more during the night. Late dinners or heavy evening snacks may also disrupt rest. Aim to finish dinner a few hours before bed and avoid meals that are high in fat or spice. If you're hungry before bed, choose something light and easy to digest.

Tobacco can make sleep problems worse. Nicotine is a stimulant, and being around second-hand smoke has been linked to disrupted sleep. Avoiding both smoking and smoke exposure, especially in the evening, can lead to more restful nights. Creating a mental link between your bed and sleep can help you fall asleep faster. Try to reserve your bed for sleep and sex only. Spending too much time in bed doing other things like watching TV or scrolling on your phone may confuse that connection. If you've been lying in bed for about twenty minutes and still can't fall asleep, get up and do something relaxing in low light. Avoid checking the time or picking up your phone. Return to bed when you feel sleepy again.

Keeping track of your sleep patterns with a journal can help you spot habits or choices that affect your rest. If you're testing new routines, writing things down can give you a clearer picture of what's helping and what's not. Some people turn to supplements to support better rest. Melatonin is a common one that may help with falling asleep, and others use options like valerian, chamomile, or glycine. Since these aren't heavily regulated by the FDA, it's important to be careful about where you buy them and speak to your doctor before using anything new. And if nothing seems to help, or your sleep problems are starting to affect your health or daily life, it's worth talking to a medical professional. A doctor can check for anything more serious and help guide you toward options that suit your personal needs.

Exercise and Skin Health

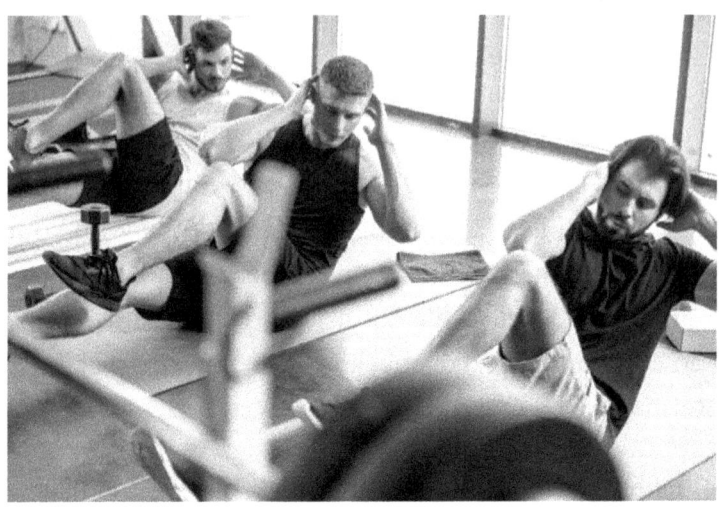

Some people assume that working out harms their skin because of the sweat it produces. But this isn't always true. There are plenty of simple ways to care for your skin while staying active, making it possible to enjoy both the physical and skin-related benefits that exercise can offer.

Physical activity supports overall wellness, and this includes the condition of your skin. One of the most noticeable effects of movement is increased circulation. As the heart pumps faster, blood moves more efficiently throughout the body. This better flow delivers important nutrients and oxygen to your skin, which supports repair and encourages cell turnover. With enough oxygen reaching the surface, skin tends to look more refreshed and full of life.

Another benefit of exercise is its role in helping the body release unwanted waste. Harmful substances from things like pollution, excess sugar, sun exposure, and tobacco can affect the skin over time. They may lead to irritation, blemishes, or visible aging. Staying active helps support circulation and the lymphatic system, which are both involved in flushing these harmful elements out of the body. When your system is functioning well, it's easier to protect your skin from damage.

Stress is a major factor that often shows up on the face. Long-term stress can make skin conditions like acne, rosacea, or eczema more difficult to manage. Physical activity encourages the release of hormones that lift your mood, helping to calm tension and reduce anxiety. It also brings cortisol levels down. Since cortisol is known to interfere with the immune system, having lower amounts makes it easier for the body to protect and restore the skin.

Maintaining a youthful look also depends on how your body handles everyday pressures. Working out regularly can support better sleep, which plays a major part in how your skin heals and stays firm. Getting enough rest helps the body repair itself, including the skin. Just half an hour of aerobic movement a few times a week has been linked to a more youthful appearance. With the right routine, you can support your skin and enjoy all the benefits of staying active.

Preventing Post-Workout Breakouts

Before starting your workout, it's a good idea to remove any makeup. Physical activity increases circulation, which opens up the pores. When makeup mixes with sweat and bacteria, it can become trapped in the skin and eventually block pores, leading to breakouts. Keeping the face clean beforehand helps minimize this risk. If your hair is long, pulling it away from your face is another smart step. Hair products and natural oils can transfer onto your skin, which may contribute to clogged pores or irritation. Hair can also trap sweat against your face, which may create an environment where unwanted bacteria or yeast can grow, causing skin problems.

Anything that touches your face while you exercise should be clean. Whether it's headphones, glasses, or helmet straps, wiping them down before use helps prevent the transfer of dirt, oil, and bacteria. This also applies to shared gym gear. Although most people clean equipment after use, it's best not to assume. Giving surfaces a quick wipe before you start will help avoid skin contact with grime or other buildup left behind by someone else. Try not to touch your face while working out. Any dirt, oil, or bacteria on your hands can transfer directly to your skin. This habit often goes unnoticed but can lead to blocked pores or irritation over time.

Wear clothing that allows your skin to breathe. Tight, sweaty clothes can trap heat and moisture, creating the perfect setting for breakouts. Certain types of acne, particularly fungal ones caused by yeast, may appear under these conditions and are often mistaken for bacterial acne. This type of skin concern often requires a specific treatment approach and won't respond to typical acne products. After your workout, change into clean, dry clothes as soon as possible. Leaving damp clothes on for too long can allow bacteria and sweat to linger against the skin, increasing the risk of irritation or blemishes. Washing your workout gear before wearing it again is also important, as sweat and oils can remain in the fabric.

When possible, take a shower after exercising. This helps remove anything that may have built up on your skin—sweat, bacteria, oil, and dirt. For those prone to acne, a cleanser with benzoyl peroxide may help by reducing the bacteria that contribute to breakouts. If this feels too drying or strong, go for a gentler, oil-free cleanser or micellar water to refresh the skin until you can shower fully. If you can't bathe right away, at the very least wash your face. Adding a retinoid to your routine can also support clearer skin. These vitamin A-based products encourage skin cell turnover and can help clean out pores. Adapalene, available without a prescription, can be useful for managing mild to moderate acne. For more persistent cases, a healthcare provider might recommend something stronger.

Carry a clean towel with you each time you work out. While towels are helpful for dabbing away sweat, they can also trap bacteria if not cleaned properly. Choose one that's soft and quick to dry, and avoid reusing the same one without washing it first. Keeping your towel fresh ensures that you aren't unintentionally spreading sweat or bacteria back onto your skin.

Chapter Sixteen

Skincare on a Budget and When to Splurge

When it comes to caring for your skin without spending a fortune, there are several dependable options that do the job well. Keeping things simple and budget-friendly doesn't mean sacrificing quality. A gentle cleansing routine is the first step. Options like Dove bar soap, Face Facts cleanser, Simple face cleanser, and Beauty Formulas face wash are easy to find and kind to the skin. For those looking for something more specialized, CeraVe face wash and the Skin1002 Madagascar Centella foam offer mild yet effective cleansing without drying the skin. Toning helps refresh the skin after cleansing. Basic choices like rose water or toners from Face Facts, Simple, and Beauty Formulas are great for everyday use. If you're looking to try something a little different, ANUA's Heartleaf mini toner is a compact and gentle option for soothing the skin.

Hydration is just as important, whether for the face or the rest of the body. Face Facts, Simple hydrating light moisturizer, and Beauty Formulas all offer face creams that lock in moisture without feeling greasy. For body care, Vaseline Healthy Bright Gluta lotion, Teals probiotic lemon balm lotion, and Face Facts ceramide body lotion all deliver good hydration and are suitable for daily use. Sun protection is something no skincare routine should skip. Tiam B3 niacin sunscreen, Biore UV Aqua Rich, and TOCOBO's calming sun serum all provide strong coverage without being heavy or chalky on the skin. They're great for daily use, especially in hot or humid climates.

Gentle exfoliation is useful to help the skin shed dead cells and stay smooth. The Face Facts mango butter scrub and Dove's Glow Recharge body scrub both offer a soft polish without causing irritation. If you like keeping things natural and homemade, mixing sugar and honey creates a simple scrub that can leave your skin feeling soft and refreshed. Affordable skincare doesn't have to be complicated. A consistent routine using trusted, wallet-friendly products can go a long way in maintaining healthy, clean, and smooth skin.

Affordable Drugstore Brands

Although recent trends suggest that many women are stepping away from daily makeup routines, especially after the global health crisis, there's still steady movement in the beauty industry. According to Thinknum, beauty products continue to draw attention, particularly in well-known stores like Target and Walgreens. Brands that already have a wide presence appear to be maintaining strong customer interest.

At Target, several names have remained popular with shoppers. Burt's Bees continues to be a go-to for natural beauty solutions. Maybelline and e.l.f. are both well-loved for their variety and affordability. Sonia Kashuk offers tools and accessories that blend well with both beginner and experienced makeup routines. Haircare brands like Pantene and skincare staples such as Dove Beauty are also high on the list. Yes To, SheaMoisture, and Pacifica bring plant-based choices into the mix, while L'Oreal, Covergirl, NYX, and Olay remain household staples across various product categories. Aveeno rounds out the list with a strong reputation in gentle skincare.

At Walgreens, a similar pattern is visible with some differences. Olay, L'Oreal, and Neutrogena continue to perform well due to their wide range of products and skin-focused solutions. Makeup favorites like Maybelline, Covergirl, NYX, and Revlon remain steady in consumer choices. Rimmel and Wet n Wild offer budget-friendly selections that appeal to many. Soap & Glory adds a bit of fun to body care, while No7 is appreciated for its skincare collections. Aveeno and SheaMoisture also appear on this list, reinforcing their popularity across multiple retailers. Burt's Bees once again makes an appearance, speaking to its strong consumer loyalty. Even with shifts in routines, it's clear that trusted beauty names still hold strong appeal.

Multi-Use Products

Products that serve more than one purpose can help simplify your routine while saving both time and space. Items like beauty balms can provide light coverage while moisturizing the skin. Concealers can double as a quick fix for uneven tone or blemishes and can be used in place of foundation when you want a lighter finish. Coconut oil is often used for multiple needs, from removing makeup to hydrating dry areas. Moisturizing creams can act as both a day and night cream, depending on your skin type and needs. Some cleansers are designed to remove makeup and also clean the skin deeply, reducing the need for multiple steps. Toners that hydrate can also calm irritation, while certain serums can be used for both brightening and smoothing. Sunscreens now often come with extra care benefits like anti-aging or hydration. A gentle cleansing gel might also work well as a shaving aid. Eye creams, though targeted, can sometimes be used around the lip area to soften lines. Facial masks that contain clay or calming ingredients might serve as spot treatments when applied directly to troubled areas. Choosing items that do more than one thing keeps your routine practical and easy to manage.

When to Splurge

When it comes to skincare, there are times when spending a bit more makes sense, especially on products that deliver results with consistent use. Items like SkinCeuticals Soothing Cleanser, Cetaphil Daily Facial Cleanser, and L'Oréal Paris Age Perfect Day Cream with SPF are known for their quality and skin-friendly formulas. Olay Regenerist Micro-Sculpting Cream, Aveeno Moisturizer Gel, and Anew Ultimate Night Cream offer added care for hydration, texture improvement, and firmness. Clinique's Moisturizing Lotion+, Kiehl's Ultra Facial Cream, and Olay's Retinol 24 line are other top choices when aiming for better skin texture and tone. These products may cost more than basic drugstore options, but their performance often justifies the price.

When considering cosmetic treatments, it's smart to compare pricing in your area. Injectable treatments like BOTOX® Cosmetic and JUVÉDERM® usually have base rates shared by the manufacturers. Knowing the average charges around you can help you decide which treatments and providers fall within your budget. Still, price isn't the only factor to consider. The skills and background of the person offering the service, along with the cleanliness of the facility and the tools used, matter a lot. Getting your treatment from a trained professional in a clean, well-run space helps protect your health and improves your chances of a good result.

Many practices offer ways to save without sacrificing quality. Clinics often have loyalty programs where repeat visits lead to better pricing or special access to deals. Some even have monthly offers just for registered clients. You may also find bundled services offered at reduced rates when you commit to more than one session at a time. For those using services from Allergan Aesthetics—makers of JUVÉDERM®, BOTOX® Cosmetic, CoolSculpting®, and Kybella®—there's a rewards system called Allē. This program gives you points for qualifying purchases, which you can later use to get discounts on future treatments. Even better, you can sometimes use these rewards along with other clinic discounts for added savings. Keeping track of these programs can make your skincare routine easier on your wallet while still allowing you to access quality treatments.

Chapter Seventeen

Simplifying Your Routine

Minimalist skincare, often called skinimalism, is all about keeping things simple and choosing only the products that matter most. It moves away from the clutter of overly complex routines and focuses instead on fewer items made with quality ingredients. The approach favors clarity and balance over layering too many formulas, which can sometimes overwhelm the skin and lead to irritation. When creating a routine that works best for your skin, sticking with what has consistently delivered good results can be more effective than constantly switching between the latest trends.

Finding the right set of products might take a bit of experimenting, especially when figuring out what works well with your specific skin needs. Still, once you land on the right mix, the payoff can be worth the effort. Minimalism in skincare doesn't mean giving up results—it means streamlining to avoid unnecessary steps while supporting your skin in the best way possible. By focusing only on what's necessary, you can keep your skin routine manageable and see long-term improvement in both comfort and appearance. Over time, your skin can start to look and feel better without the extra stress that sometimes comes from too many active ingredients.

The Rise of Minimal Skincare

In a world where everything seems to come with too many choices—from what to watch online to what to eat in the morning—it's no surprise that skincare shelves are equally overwhelming. Dozens of serums, masks, toners, and exfoliants promise flawless skin, making it easy to feel like you need a 10-step routine just to keep up. But amid the noise, a refreshing shift has quietly gained traction: the return to simple, scaled-back skincare.

Part of this shift is rooted in a growing awareness of how sensitive skin can be. More people are paying attention to conditions like eczema, rosacea, and persistent breakouts, and realizing that overloading the skin with too many active ingredients often does more harm than good. A minimal routine gives the skin room to recover, using just a few targeted products that meet its specific needs without piling on layers of unnecessary formulas.

At the same time, people are leaning into a more thoughtful, science-supported approach. Dermatologists frequently recommend focusing on just a few daily habits: cleansing, moisturizing, and using sunscreen. These simple steps can do a lot of the heavy lifting when it comes to keeping your skin clear, balanced, and protected. For many, sticking with the basics has led to clearer, calmer skin and a far easier routine to maintain.

There's also a growing concern about the impact of personal care products on the planet. With beauty packaging often made from plastic and used only briefly, the environmental cost is adding up. By paring down the number of products, minimal skincare not only reduces waste but also makes it easier to support brands that offer better choices in how they produce and package what we use.

At its core, minimal skincare means choosing a few products that serve multiple purposes. It might mean using a cleanser that also hydrates or a moisturizer that includes SPF. It's about paying attention to how your skin reacts, understanding what it really needs, and letting that guide your choices. Fewer steps also mean it's easier to stick with your routine, which helps your skin settle into a rhythm. People who've embraced this approach find that their skin becomes more balanced, easier to manage, and less prone to sudden changes. The idea that less can truly do more is proving to be not just practical but effective.

Benefits of Minimalist Skincare Routines

Choosing a minimalist approach to skincare has become more common as users try to simplify their routines and reduce unnecessary waste. While it may seem counterintuitive in a market full of tempting new releases, cutting back on the number of products you use can actually be quite effective. The idea is to focus only on a few essentials and use them consistently. This not only helps reduce clutter but can also improve your skin's condition in the long run.

One of the most noticeable benefits is how much time you save. With fewer steps to go through, your skincare process becomes quicker and easier to follow. Instead of juggling multiple layers morning and night, you stick to the basics, which makes daily care feel less like a chore and more like a habit you can manage even on the busiest days. Minimal routines also tend to be easier on the wallet. Rather than buying a wide range of products that may or may not work for you, focusing on a few well-formulated items allows you to invest in better quality without overspending. Over time, this can cut down on the cost of replacing ineffective or unused products.

There's also the benefit of a cleaner, more organized space. When you reduce the number of items in your bathroom or on your vanity, it's easier to keep everything neat. You avoid the pile-up of half-used jars and bottles and make room for what really matters. For those with sensitive skin, a scaled-back routine often brings welcome relief. Fewer products mean fewer chances for your skin to come into contact with ingredients that might cause irritation. When something does trigger a reaction, it's easier to identify the cause because your routine is simple and focused. This type of routine is much easier to maintain. With a busy schedule, it's hard to keep up with ten different products every day. A short list of reliable go-tos makes it easier to stay consistent, and it's often that regularity—not the number of products—that leads to real results over time. Simplicity, in this case, can be just what your skin needs.

Keeping your skincare routine simple is a great way to avoid overwhelming your skin with too many products. Start by focusing on the essentials—just a cleanser, moisturizer, and sunscreen can go a long way. If your skin can tolerate it, adding a toner or serum may offer added support, but they aren't always necessary for everyone. Choosing products that serve more than one purpose is another smart move. A good example is a moisturizer that also contains SPF, which cuts down on the number of layers you apply while still protecting and hydrating your skin.

Be mindful of how often you exfoliate. While exfoliation helps remove dead skin and smooth texture, doing it too frequently can leave your skin dry, irritated, or prone to breakouts. Twice a week is often enough for most people, but this can vary depending on your skin's sensitivity.

If you're unsure what your skin needs or which products to stick with, it's a good idea to speak with a skincare professional. They can help you figure out what suits your skin best so you don't end up using unnecessary products that could cause more harm than good. Keeping things simple and focused can help your skin stay calm, balanced, and healthy over time.

Chapter Eighteen

Skincare Routine for Men

Skincare isn't something that should be limited to women—it's an important part of daily care for everyone. Men's skin also faces daily stress from the environment, shaving, and buildup of oil or dirt. Taking time to care for your skin is not about luxury; it's about maintaining good hygiene, comfort, and confidence. Unfortunately, there's still an outdated belief that skincare is only for women, which keeps many men from building routines that actually benefit them. It's time to move past that idea and treat skincare for what it really is—basic maintenance that keeps your skin clear, smooth, and refreshed, regardless of gender.

Men's skin tends to be thicker and can produce more oil than women's, which means it may be more prone to breakouts and irritation. Daily exposure to things like dust, sun, and pollution also takes a toll, often without being noticed until signs show up. Taking care of your skin isn't about keeping up appearances—it's about maintaining its strength and function. A good routine helps protect against clogged pores, dryness, sun damage, and other problems that can build up over time if left unchecked. Regular care gives your skin the support it needs to stay clear and steady through everyday stress.

Common Skincare Issues for Men

Men often face their own set of skin-related concerns, including irritation from shaving, ingrown hairs, and increased sun exposure from regularly removing facial hair. These challenges call for a routine that's tailored to handle those effects. Razor burn, for example, can be soothed with gentle shaving techniques and products that calm the skin afterward. Having a collection of daily-use items makes the process more manageable while keeping the skin in good condition.

Essentials might include body sunscreen, a mild facial cleanser, toner, and a daytime moisturizer that has built-in SPF or antioxidant support. For nighttime, a moisturizer with retinol can help with skin renewal. Eye cream, lip balm, and a light hand lotion support smaller, sensitive areas. Spot treatments like blemish gel can help control occasional breakouts. Keeping clean with shower gel and staying fresh with antiperspirant are part of the mix too, along with a preferred cologne and shaving foam that doesn't irritate. Each of these steps works together to keep the skin balanced and well-cared for, without needing an overwhelming number of products.

Addressing Unique Skin Concerns

Forehead lines are a common concern, especially as the skin begins to change with time. They're a natural part of getting older, often forming as skin loses its stretch and firmness. Still, some people prefer to include products in their routine that may help reduce how noticeable those lines become. One ingredient often used for this purpose is retinol, a form of vitamin A. It's found in a variety of over-the-counter and prescription skincare items and has been known to support smoother-looking skin when used consistently. By encouraging skin renewal, it can play a role in softening the look of lines and bringing a more even feel to the surface over time.

Blackheads are one of the most common blemishes and show up when excess oil and dead skin block the pores. They're dark in appearance—hence the name—and are often called open comedones. While it may be tempting to press or squeeze them, doing so can push bacteria deeper and cause more breakouts, discoloration, or even lasting marks. Instead, it's better to follow a routine that targets clogged pores, exfoliate regularly, and stick to products labeled as non-comedogenic, which means they won't block your pores.

If you've noticed tiny black dots on your nose, they might not be blackheads at all. They could be sebaceous filaments, which are more common in oily skin. These occur when oil and dead skin collect in a pore, but they don't clog it. While they can't be removed entirely, sticking to a consistent routine that includes exfoliation can reduce how noticeable they look.

Razor bumps, which often show up as red, irritated spots after shaving, can cause discomfort. These bumps can appear on the face, underarms, or anywhere a razor is used. Prepping your skin before shaving—like using exfoliators, applying shaving gel, and shaving in the direction of hair growth—can help reduce them.

While your skin needs natural oils to stay balanced, too much can leave it looking greasy. Managing excess shine starts with finding a cleanser that matches your skin type and gently washes away buildup without stripping it dry.

Large pores are another concern, especially for those with oilier skin. They may also become more visible as you age. Though pore size can't be changed, there are steps you can take to reduce how noticeable they appear.

Skin that feels rough or looks dull often hasn't been exfoliated enough. Buildup of dead skin cells can affect both appearance and texture. Instead of rough scrubs, go for something like a chemical exfoliant with glycolic acid. It's easier to add to a daily routine and tends to be gentler on the skin.

If your skin lacks a fresh or healthy glow, buildup of old skin cells could be the reason. A simple way to restore brightness is through regular exfoliation and by using a product that contains vitamin C. Over time, this can support a more refreshed appearance.

Redness on the face can come from a number of reasons, including skin sensitivity or conditions like rosacea. If it's something that happens often, it's a good idea to talk to a skincare professional. While waiting for a clear answer, color-correcting products with green tones can help even things out.

Dry skin is something almost everyone experiences at some point. Whether caused by weather, environment, or your skin type, regular moisturizing helps restore comfort and appearance. It also supports the skin's ability to stay soft and smooth.

Hyperpigmentation refers to dark spots or uneven skin tone. These patches can show up for many reasons. Using exfoliators as part of your routine can help create a more even surface. You might also try switching out your regular serum for one aimed at targeting discoloration.

Age spots—also called liver spots—are small dark patches that come from too much sun over time. The best way to help keep them from appearing is by using sunscreen every day, even when inside or on cloudy days.

Dark spots may result from past acne or sun exposure. They can take a while to fade, but using the right products—like a brightening treatment or face peel—can help over time. Spot correctors are a great addition to your daily routine if you're trying to even out your skin tone.

Fine lines under the eyes are common as skin matures. One way to treat this is by applying a gentle product made for the eye area. This step can support smoother-looking skin with regular use.

Puffiness around the eyes can be caused by a lack of rest. Though different from under-eye bags, which often run in families, this temporary swelling can be managed with products made specifically for that area. They help give the skin a more rested look.

Dark circles don't always mean you're sleep-deprived. They can show up because of age, heredity, or lifestyle. Still, a tired night can make them more obvious. Adding a brightening eye cream or serum can help soften their appearance and give your under-eyes a more refreshed look.

Simplify the Routine

Keeping your skincare routine simple can be one of the best ways to keep your skin happy as a man. By sticking to the essentials, picking products that serve more than one purpose, and staying aware of how your skin responds, you can build a plan that's both practical and effective. Start with the foundation of any routine—cleansing, moisturizing, and sun protection. A gentle face wash helps clear away buildup without stripping your skin. After that, a lightweight moisturizer keeps your skin soft and balanced throughout the day. To finish, apply a sunscreen with SPF 30 or higher to defend against sun exposure.

Choosing products that serve multiple functions can also help you streamline things. For instance, some moisturizers or makeup items come with sun protection built in. Others offer hydration while addressing specific concerns like dullness or uneven texture. Fewer products don't mean less care—it just means being selective with what you use.

Paying attention to your skin's behavior is key. If something starts to cause discomfort or breakouts, switch it out. Everyone's skin has different needs, and what works for someone else might not work for you. Keep it simple and adjust only when necessary. You might still want to include a few extras in your routine, depending on your skin goals. A serum with targeted ingredients can help manage concerns like dryness or uneven tone. Exfoliating once or twice a week can smooth the surface and bring a natural glow. For those with dry skin, a nourishing face oil can provide added moisture. If you're dealing with occasional blemishes, a spot treatment can help address them quickly.

Simplifying your skincare doesn't mean skipping care—it means trimming the excess. Fewer steps save time and reduce the number of products you go through, which also helps cut back on spending and waste. Thoughtful choices and consistency often lead to better results than using a shelf full of products.

Final Thoughts

Loving your skin means more than simply applying products—it's about building a kind relationship with the face you see in the mirror every day. Accepting the changes your skin goes through, from breakouts to dry patches or signs of age, is part of growing with it. Everyone's skin tells a different story, and no one's journey is the same. Instead of comparing it to someone else's, the focus should be on care, patience and understanding what your skin needs at every stage of life.

A helpful place to begin is with a gentle mindset. When your skin isn't looking its best, it's easy to be harsh with yourself. Try speaking kindly to yourself instead. Remember, your skin has a job—it protects you daily and deserves to be treated with care. Like any other part of your body, it needs rest, nourishment and time to adjust to changes. Look at what you like about your skin. It could be its tone, softness, freckles, or a warm glow in the sunlight. Shifting attention to what you appreciate rather than what bothers you can help you see yourself in a softer light.

Expecting instant results from products often leads to frustration. Skin changes slowly, and building habits that support it takes time. Progress might not be noticeable at first, but small improvements add up. Getting familiar with your skin's type and tendencies will make it easier to choose the right routine. Learn how different ingredients affect you. Whether you're dry, oily or sensitive, finding what works for you helps prevent waste and disappointment.

Whatever you use—cleanser, moisturizer, or treatment—what matters most is keeping up with it. Routines that match your skin's needs work best when done regularly. This steady approach gives your skin a better chance to adjust and recover.

If something seems off or persistent problems appear, it's a good idea to speak to a skincare professional. They can look closely at your skin and recommend products or treatments that are suitable. Their advice might also help prevent trial-and-error frustration. It also helps to be thankful for what your skin does. It holds you together, keeps out germs, and renews itself. Thinking about all the hard work it does for you each day can change how you see it.

The messages you take in from others matter, too. Following people who promote real skin, kindness, and care over perfection can shift your mindset. Whether online or in real life, try to stay around those who lift your confidence and help you feel seen and supported. Eating well, drinking enough water, getting rest, and staying active all play a part. Your skin often reflects what's going on inside, so looking after your body supports the outside, too.

At the heart of it, learning to care for your skin is also about learning to care for yourself. Accept the texture, color, marks and changes with patience. Give yourself grace, and remember you deserve to feel good in your own skin—every single day.

Staying Consistent for Long-Term Results

Sticking to a skincare routine over time means showing up for your skin every day, using the right products in the morning and at night, and giving them enough time to do their work. With steady use, your skin can slowly respond to the care it's receiving, leading to smoother texture, even tone, and more bounce. Trends in skincare may come and go, and your skin will change with the seasons and with age, but some habits should remain steady—especially your skincare routine. Eating balanced meals, staying hydrated, getting exercise, and sticking to the same basic routine can help keep your skin looking and feeling its best.

If you're trying to keep up with your routine but find it difficult, start with a simple plan that won't take more than ten minutes. Build it into a moment that already exists in your day—like right after brushing your teeth. Choose one day to exfoliate and make it part of your schedule. Little steps can make a big difference when it comes to staying consistent.

One of the hardest parts of a skincare routine can be figuring out what products to use and when. Most people know they need a cleanser and a moisturizer. But what about retinol or exfoliants that are only needed a few nights a week? To avoid confusion, make yourself a skincare calendar. Jot down which products to use on which days, especially those that don't need daily application. That way, it's all laid out for you, and you don't have to figure it out in the moment. Some people skip their evening routine simply because they wait too long and get tired. Instead of putting it off until bedtime, start your nighttime steps earlier. If you usually go to bed at 11, aim to begin your skincare by 10. Set a reminder on your phone if it helps. You'll be less sleepy and more likely to follow through. This simple change also gives your body a signal that it's time to relax and wind down.

If you respond well to rewards, consider setting up a small system for yourself. Keep track of how often you complete your routine and treat yourself after hitting your target. It could be something small, like setting aside a little money for a fun purchase or allowing yourself time for a favorite hobby. Some people are more motivated by seeing results than by rewards. If that sounds like you, take a photo of your skin each month and compare. Subtle changes can be hard to notice in real time, but side-by-side pictures will give you a clearer view. That difference might be all the push you need to keep going.

Keeping products in sight can also be a helpful reminder. When skincare items are tucked away, it's easy to forget them. Try placing them somewhere visible, like on a small shelf or inside a nice container that matches your bathroom decor. That way, they stay top of mind and easy to reach. You don't have to go it alone. Partner with a friend who's also working on a goal. It doesn't have to be skincare—just someone with a habit they're trying to build. Check in with each other daily, and give encouragement if one of you slips. This kind of accountability can make a big difference. Skincare products can offer great support for your skin, but only if you use them regularly. Whether you're motivated by tracking your progress, treating yourself for consistency, or simply enjoying the process, the goal is the same—taking care of your skin in a way that fits your lifestyle. Keep showing up for yourself. With time and regular effort, you'll begin to notice a healthy, lasting glow.

Where to Find Reliable Skincare Resources

Looking for trusted websites to buy skincare products online in the U.S.? You're in luck. As of 2024, there are plenty of great places where you can find high-quality skincare products delivered straight to your door. Below is a rundown of ten top-rated sites that offer great selections, user-friendly platforms, and added perks that make shopping easier and more enjoyable.

Sephora continues to be one of the most recognized beauty stores across the country. It offers a broad mix of skincare lines, including some brands you won't find anywhere else. Whether you're after moisturizers, cleansers, serums, or masks, you'll find plenty to pick from. The site features customer reviews to help guide your choices, and its loyalty program rewards you with points on every purchase, which can be used toward samples or future products. Plus, they regularly offer deals and free shipping over a minimum spend.

Ulta Beauty is another reliable destination. The main appeal here is the range—you'll find both luxury and drugstore labels side by side. Ulta's reward system lets you earn points for discounts later, and they often run sales that make skincare more affordable. If there's a location nearby, you can even shop online and pick up in-store. Their website is easy to navigate, and their return policy is also very flexible.

Dermstore focuses on skincare and haircare, offering products often recommended by professionals. You'll find everything from gentle cleansers to science-backed treatments. They also provide helpful articles, ingredient breakdowns, and a loyalty system where points can be used toward future purchases. If there are items you regularly use, you can opt for auto-delivery so you never run out.

SkinStore has a wide international selection, showcasing skincare from Europe, Asia, and beyond. This makes it a good place to discover new favorites. Their regular discount codes and bundled savings make it more affordable to try out multiple products at once. They also include detailed product pages and tips from skincare professionals.

Glossier focuses only on its own product line, but its clean and simple approach has won many fans. Their items are designed to be effective and easy to use. Prices are moderate, and the brand is known for its gentle ingredients and attractive packaging. The site is well-designed, making it easy to find what you're looking for and learn how to use it.

Credo Beauty is perfect for shoppers who prefer clean, non-toxic skincare. They carry a wide variety of natural brands, all held to strict safety standards. The site also educates shoppers about ingredient safety and product benefits. In-store locations are available in select areas for those who like to browse in person. Credo often includes free samples with purchases and offers items in eco-friendly packaging.

The Ordinary has become widely known for its simple approach and low prices. Most items cost less than $10 and focus on single active ingredients, letting you customize your skincare based on your needs. Though their scientific product names can be overwhelming at first, they offer guides to help you find what suits your skin. Their formulas are minimal but effective, and the brand is cruelty-free.

Paula's Choice stands out for being backed by solid research and reliable formulas. Products are designed for specific skin concerns, and their website includes tools and quizzes to guide your selection. All items come with full ingredient lists, and the brand does not use added fragrance, which is helpful for sensitive skin. If you're not satisfied, returns are accepted within 60 days.

Beautylish features a carefully picked mix of high-end skincare brands. What sets it apart is the attention to detail—the product descriptions are thorough, and you'll find customer reviews along with photos. If you're making a larger purchase, payment plans are available. The site is visually appealing, and their customer support receives strong praise.

Bluemercury focuses on upscale skincare and beauty. The shopping experience feels more like browsing a luxury spa, with expert suggestions and elegant product presentation. Orders often come with free gifts, and their rewards system allows you to collect points with every order. Physical store locations are available in some areas, giving you the option to shop in person.

Each of these websites offers something a little different, whether it's exclusive brands, affordable prices, natural options, or premium service. Depending on your budget and skincare goals, any of them could be a great place to find the right products for your needs.

Appendices
Glossary of Skincare Terms

Acne: Blemishes that appear when pores become clogged by blocked skin cells, sebum, germs and other impurities. There are many levels of severity, ranging from whiteheads and blackheads to cystic acne.

Anti-Aging: A word used to describe how a routine or product can help slow the apparent indications of aging, often known as 'photo-aging': looser skin, fine lines, wrinkles and so on.

Blackheads: These are 'open' comedones whose heads break the skin's surface and corrode to a dark color.

Broad Spectrum: This is a sunscreen that shields against two kinds of ultraviolet (UV) rays: UVA and UVB.

Combination Skin: When an individual's skin tone is a combination of oily (usually in the T-zone) and dry (usually on the cheeks).

Comedogenic: This refers to a product's ability to clog pores and produce acne (comedones).

Cystic acne: This is a deeply ingrained kind of acne, most prevalent in oily skin types. Cystic pimples are often felt before they are seen; they are usually unpleasant and should not be crushed or popped. (This will worsen the appearance and slow the healing process).

Dark Spots: Generally refers to sun spots or post-acne scars that are tough or slow to fade from the skin's surface.

Dark circles: Triggered by weariness, dehydration or aging and it refer to the region beneath the eyes where the skin is more fragile than anyplace else on the face. It is simple to look through the skin to the blood vessels on the opposite side.

Dry Skin: The state of having consistently dry/non-oily skin. Seasonal or transient dryness can develop in persons who are not accustomed to it.

Free radicals: These are atoms with an unpaired electron that can break DNA, boosting the risk of skin cancer or accelerating photoaging. Effectively prevented with antioxidant-rich products.

Hyperpigmentation: This is the darkening of large sections of skin caused by an unexpected rise in melanin as a result of sun exposure, irritation or medical conditions.

K-Beauty / K-Grooming: This refers to the global trend of ingredients- and routine-focused skincare. The typical K-Beauty routine consists of ten phases, which can be changed (up or down) to meet the demands of each individual.

Normal Skin: This refers to skin that is neither overly oily nor dry. This would be the best "balanced" skin type.

Oily Skin: A skin condition characterized by excessive sebum generation. This also makes you more susceptible to acne.

pH: This is a scale of 0-14 that indicates how acidic or basicity something is. Pure water has a pH of 7 and anything beneath it is acidic, while anything higher is basic/alkaline. (pH means 'potential of hydrogen'.) In skincare, we compare a product's pH level to that of skin, which is somewhat acidic (at 4.7-5.75). The goal is to keep the skin in this range of pH levels after using treatments so that it does not become too dry or irritated.

Photoaging: This is when the skin reveals visible indications of aging. Exposure to pollutants and ultraviolet radiation can accelerate the process, but a proactive anti-aging program combined with a healthy lifestyle and frequent SPF use can slow it down.

Pores: These are microscopic surface holes on the skin that discharge sweat and oil. Individuals with oily skin typically have larger pores. Acne occurs when pores become congested or clogged with bacteria, dead skin cells, sebum and other substances.

Razor Bumps: This refers to the painful, unattractive irritation that occurs after shaving when hairs get caught under the skin.

Sebum: This refers to the "oil" produced by the skin that naturally moisturizes and conditions the skin and hair. Excessive sebum production can make you appear and feel oily, as well as block your pores. However, the production of sebum, in general, is essential for overall skin health.

T-Zone: The "T" shape formed by the forehead and nose (sometimes including the chin). The T-Zone is frequently mentioned when talking about oil patterns or acne accumulation on the skin, as it is oilier than other regions of the face.

UVA Rays: This refers to the ultraviolet rays that seep deep into the skin and speed up photoaging.

UVB Rays: This refers to the (UV) rays that lead to sunburn and can boost the risk of melanoma/skin cancer.

Whiteheads: These are 'closed' or locked comedones that form beneath the skin, but the head turns white because of the pressure of trapped dirt.

SKIN TERMS/CONCERNS

Acmella Oleracea: This is a plant extract that relaxes facial muscles and minimizes the visibility of wrinkles and fine lines.

Alpha Hydroxy Acids: AHAs like glycolic, lactic and citric acids, which help remove dead surface cells and create a brighter, more velvety and more even skin tone.

Amino acids: These are the "building blocks" of proteins that assist the skin in forming keratin, elastic collagen and other proteins and, as a result, keep the skin firm and elastic.

Antioxidants: These are the fighters of free radicals, pollutants and ultraviolet radiation that cause skin aging. An antioxidant-rich skincare routine prevents these items from reaching the skin's surface.

Argan Oil: A highly nourishing, not acne-causing oil that is often used in skin and hair care products. High in Vitamin E.

Barley Extract: This is an antioxidant-rich component that also enhances hydration and suppleness.

Beta Hydroxy Acid: BHAs, most commonly salicylic acid, aid in the elimination of dead skin cells and sebum locked inside the pores. This can help treat and control acne.

Cactus Extract: This is a calming, moisturizing and firming component. Cactus extract also contains linoleic acid, which aids in the regulation of sebum levels in the skin.

Ceramides: This strengthens the skin's barrier functions by retaining moisture within the skin and establishing a defense against pollutants, toxins and other contaminants.

Charcoal: Known for its cleansing and detoxifying properties, charcoal is used in both cleansing and moisturizing items (products).

Cica: Also referred to as Tiger Grass, it is incredibly calming and can treat minor irritation as well as more serious conditions such as eczema or psoriasis.

Clay: Has the highest absorbent power of any cleansing component. Usually found in facial masks and cleansers to help remove excess sebum, dirt and pollutants from the pores.

Collagen: This is the protein that serves as the foundation for our skin and body. Collagen helps to make our skin firmer and suppler. As we grow older, our bodies create less collagen, which causes looser skin.

Emollient: Topical products that create a layer on top of the skin, such as moisturizers and oils. These items should be used last in a skincare routine (since other products will not likely penetrate them). They can aid in keeping moisture levels in the skin.

Glycerin: This is a typical humectant component in skincare that helps draw moisture into the skin.

Haloxyl: This is a patented peptide-powered compound that helps reduce the visibility of dark circles beneath the eyes.

Heartleaf (Houttuynia cordata): Heartleaf is antimicrobial and anti-inflammatory, making it a soothing complement to any skincare routine and is particularly useful for sensitive skin.

Humectants: These are skincare products that are rubbed on the skin to attract moisture from the surrounding air (such as glycerin and hyaluronic acid). They are preferable for persons with dry skin who require additional moisture but are best avoided during dry months because humectants can make up for a lack of moisture in the air by drawing hydration from deeper inside the skin.

Hyaluronic Acid: A humectant component that can absorb moisture from the air and retain up to 1,000 times its own weight in water.

Jojoba Oil: This is a non-comedogenic, ultra-moisturizing ingredient that is excellent for all skin types.

Kaolin: This is a typical kind of clay used in thorough cleaning, purifying masks and cleansers.

Niacinamide: A powerful smoother, niacinamide enhances skin surface texture and look; it can minimize the visibility of dullness, pores, hyperpigmentation, fine lines, dark spots, rough patches and other skin imperfections.

Oat Extract: A calming and nourishing component that is especially useful for dry skin.

Peptides: These are amino acids that act as the basis for protein in the skin (this helps in the generation of keratin, elastin and collagen).

Polyhydroxy Acid: PHAs (such as galactose, gluconolactone and lactobionic acid) aid in the removal of dead surface cells, although they do not penetrate as deeply as AHAs. They are generally milder, as AHAs can leave skin more prone to things like sunshine.

Prickly Pear Cactus: Anti-inflammatory and relaxing, prickly pear cactus calms and nourishes all skin types.

Retinoids and retinol: These are vitamin A compounds that have been shown to reverse and greatly slow photoaging. It can be found over the counter in lesser quantities or prescription in greater concentrations (usually as tretinoin).

Rosehip Oil: Extremely nourishing and firming for your skin. High in fatty acids and linoleic acid, which helps to tone the skin.

Salicylic Acid: The most prevalent form of beta hydroxy acid (BHA), it helps to clear pores and prevent acne.

SPF: "Sun Protection Factor"; SPF is a product's capacity to protect skin from the sun's ultraviolet radiation. The SPF value on a product indicates how long you may stay in the sun without burning. (SPF 15 is 15x longer, for instance). However, SPF should be applied again every two hours while in the sun, as well as after swimming or sweating.

Vitamin A: This helps to reduce acne and enhances surface texture while reducing and reversing the symptoms of photoaging.

Vitamin B3: B3 (niacinamide) enhances surface texture and look. B12 promotes cellular metabolism and hastens renewal (which reduces dark spots and accelerates healing), as well as firming the skin.

Vitamin C: This is a potent antioxidant that helps to stop aging and brightens the appearance of the skin.

Vitamin D: This can be synthesized with adequate (healthy) sun exposure. It is anti-inflammatory and can neutralize free radicals. (Just remember to use SPF to avoid Ultraviolet damage to your skin.)

Vitamin E: Aids strengthen the skin's barrier functions and is an excellent antioxidant.

Vitamin K: Helps to stimulate collagen formation in the skin, which can speed up wound healing.

KEY PRODUCTS

Cleanser: This removes dirt, filth, oil and other impurities from the skin's surface. As the initial step in your skincare program, apply two times a day (morning and night).

Cleansing/Detox Mask: This can be utilized once a week to eliminate excess sebum and dirt from deep inside the pores.

Concealer: A dense, skin-toned cream that conceals minor imperfections such as acne, dark circles and redness.

Essence: Lightweight sprays that can heal or nourish the skin (based on the formula). Generally applied after cleanser but prior to serums and moisturizers.

Exfoliator: A physical scrub or chemical substance that aids in the elimination of dead surface skin cells, hence preventing clogged pores and sallowness.

Eye Cream: An aimed cream (or serum) specifically designed for the region around the eyes, which is specifically prone to puffiness, dark circles and photoaging. Eye creams are frequently formulated with skin-firming peptides or circulation-enhancing caffeine.

Hydrating/Deep Nourishing Mask: A mask that can be left on or applied overnight to nourish the skin profoundly. It can be utilized every couple of days or once per week to augment a current hydration routine. (Best worn overnight.)

Moisturizer: An essential skincare phase, moisturizer enriches the skin while also stopping moisture loss by protecting it with its emollient properties. Daytime moisturizers frequently incorporate SPF.

Night Cream: A bedtime moisturizer that's usually more concentrated with ingredients (compared to daytime moisturizers) and no SPF. Night creams work with the body's nighttime cellular renewal to speed up healing and maximize ingredient benefits.

Serum: A light product used after cleansers and essences but before moisturizers. Serums can either nourish profoundly (such as hyaluronic acid), exfoliate (such as glycolic acid or other AHAs) or treat/prevent disorders (such as acne/breakout-prone skin with salicylic acid).

Sheet Masks: Sheet masks are often moisturizing and contain high-concentration serums that deeply repair or treat the skin.

Spot Treatment: A product that uses neutralizing agents to target a specific blemish (such as a dark spot or breakout), as treating the entire face may be too forceful or unneeded.

Toner: This can help balance the pH of the skin between the cleanser or treatment and the hydrating/moisturizing phases. Toners can also balance oil levels and soothe skin after shaving. Avoid toners containing alcohol.

Product Recommendations by Category

When choosing skincare products, it helps to think about what your skin needs and what concerns you're trying to manage. Picking the right product depends on your skin type—whether it's dry, oily, a mix of both, or sensitive—and what you want to improve, like breakouts, fine lines, or dullness. There are many trusted products that people reach for across different steps of their skincare routine, including cleansing, moisturizing, and treating targeted concerns.

For moisture, Neutrogena's Hydro Boost Water Gel is a favorite for good reason. It feels lightweight, absorbs fast, and suits both dry and acne-prone skin. It hydrates without leaving behind a greasy film, which is a big plus for those who are worried about breakouts.

If acne is something you're managing, CeraVe's Acne Foaming Cream Cleanser is a gentle but effective option. It works to break down oil and dirt without over-drying the skin, which can sometimes happen with stronger acne cleansers.

To address early signs of aging or support overall skin texture, Cosrx Advanced Snail 96 Mucin Power Essence is a go-to for many. It's a lightweight serum that adds moisture and helps keep skin looking smooth and even-toned. It's often recommended as part of a balanced routine for aging skin.

Removing makeup can sometimes be a challenge, especially around the eyes, but The INKEY List Oat Cleansing Balm makes it easier. It gently removes makeup without irritating the skin or leaving behind residue, and it doesn't contain added oils that could clog pores.

For daily cleansing that works across skin types, **CeraVe's** Hydrating Cleanser stands out. It's mild, fragrance-free, and helps maintain your skin's natural barrier, making it a solid choice whether your skin is dry, oily, or somewhere in between.

No matter your routine, using products that suit your skin's needs and staying consistent with them can make a big difference over time. The key is to keep it simple, be patient, and let your skin tell you what works.

Frequently Asked Skincare Questions and Answers

Is it crucial to moisturize?

Yes, each skin type requires moisturizer. It helps to replenish water in your skin, which promotes the barrier function. Without sufficient moisturization, your skin will be susceptible to acne and dryness, which will boost wrinkle generation and irritation. Individuals with dry skin benefit from a thick and creamy moisturizer, while those with oily/acne-prone/combination skin should opt for a lightweight one.

Can I shrink my pores?

Pores are normal and help your skin breathe. However, you cannot 'shrink' the size or literally reduce their size. What you have the ability to do is to reduce their appearance. This will help to smooth out the look of your skin and improve your complexion significantly. Applying toner two times a day helps refine and tighten your pores.

Is it too late to begin using SPF?

It's never too late to begin using SPF and shielding your skin. Sun protection can help your skin at any age. So, it's okay to begin late instead of not beginning at all.

Is it permissible to pick spots?

No. Doing this can cause irreversible damage to your skin. Picking at hyperpigmented regions or scars breaks the skin's barrier, thus exacerbating the condition instead of alleviating it. A brightening component, such as Vitamin C or Niacinamide, will help minimize discoloration and fade the spots as time passes.

How crucial is it to wear sunscreen every day?

Putting on sunscreen every day is one of the most effective strategies to shield your skin's look and general health. When used daily, it protects your skin from sunburn, tan, premature indications of aging and even some kinds of skin cancer. You must always use it at least twenty minutes before going out in the sun.

Is it important to cleanse my face every morning and evening?

The general rule of thumb is to cleanse your face two times every day. It purifies and energizes your skin in the morning and helps to remove dirt and grime from your face in the evening. The correct cleanser will mildly cleanse your skin while preserving its natural moisture. A 100% soap-free cleanser will help you get there.

Can I wash my face with water?

You can use only water to cleanse your face after a workout or to refresh throughout the day. However, simply using water to cleanse your face instead of a face wash is not recommended.

How do I incorporate exfoliating components into my routine?

Chemical exfoliators are highly effective and can help you address certain skin conditions. With regard to this, you should only use them 1-2 times per week. It is also vital to remember that you are not to layer these components together because it can damage your skin's barrier.

How can I know my skin type?

You would begin by washing your face with a mild cleanser and carefully patting it dry. Do not use any skincare products and wait thirty to forty minutes. If your face is generally glossy, you have oily skin. If your T-zone is shiny while the remaining area of your face is normal, you have a combination skin. If your skin appears a bit tight, you have dry skin.

Should I adjust my skincare routine with every season?

Ideally, absolutely. The transitioning weather necessitates a routine that adjusts to your skin's requirements. For instance, your skin may like light formulations in the summer but require more nourishing and creamy formulas in the winter.

Should I still use moisturizer if my skin is oily skin?

Yes! Oily skin needs extra water or a moisturizing moisturizer to balance excessive sebum production. In the absence of a moisturizer, your skin will generate extra oil to compensate for the lack of water. Choose a lightweight, quick-absorbing moisturizer that matches your skin without leaving it oily.

Does drinking water truly help you get clear skin?

Taking a minimum of 2-3 liters of water per day helps eliminate toxins from the blood and helps to enhance your skin tone and general appearance.

Can I still get sunburned if I apply SPF-containing makeup?

If you spend most of the day outside and do not reapply sunscreen every two or three hours, you may become sunburned. For ongoing and best UV protection, use a broad-spectrum sunscreen with a minimal SPF of 50.

Can over-the-counter acne remedies produce the same results as prescription ones?

Over-the-counter acne therapies are efficient but far gentler than prescription medication. Because of this, they may take longer to produce benefits, but they can be utilized without a doctor's supervision.

What is Vitamin C and how does it benefit your skincare routine?

Vitamin C is a nutrient contained in the body that offers health benefits when ingested as part of a balanced diet. Several individuals utilize it topically. Vitamin C has remarkable anti-aging properties and can lower the visibility of fine lines and creases (wrinkles). Furthermore, because of its strong antioxidant qualities, it shields the skin from free radical damage. This implies that it protects against premature skin aging. Also, vitamin C promotes collagen formation, resulting in tighter, younger-looking skin overall.

How Do You Apply Retinol?

Generally, retinol is commonly used in nighttime skincare regimes. This is because this potent ingredient eliminates dead skin cells from the top layer of the skin's surface. This renders the skin more prone to sunlight damage. Furthermore, start by applying retinol three times each week and slowly increase the frequency. This is related to the potency of retinol. Slowly increasing the frequency will enable your skin to become accustomed to the product, thus reducing irritation. It's also vital to use a high-quality moisturizer after applying retinol to alleviate any dryness or irritation. Furthermore, in the morning, use SPF30+. This protects your skin from the UV damage that retinol might cause.

Does How You Sleep Influence Your Face Shape?

As time passes, sleep can alter the form and look of your skin. This is because your face is squashed into your pillow for several hours each night. Finally, this can compress the surface of your skin, causing wrinkles to appear. As a result, changing your pillows every one to two years will help to improve the support for your skin.

What should I wear first in my skincare routine: moisturizer or SPF?

Moisturizers should always be used first. As a result, this enables the moisturizer to seep into the skin before SPF is applied. SPF should also be the last step in your skincare process because it has a thicker consistency and should not overpower the thinner products.

Does SPF require to be worn indoors or when it's cloudy?

As previously stated, SPF is an essential aspect of any skincare program and should be the final step. It is particularly crucial on days when the sun isn't as harsh. Even in the winter, harmful ultraviolet (UV) Rays are able to still pass through clouds and even windows, leaving you susceptible to severe skin damage. This is particularly true if your skin isn't properly protected. Sun damage can cause dark patches, wrinkles and, in extreme circumstances, skin cancer. SPF should be used every day!

How Can You Manage Acne and Anxiety-Induced Outbreaks with Skincare?

Anxiety-inspired breakouts are fairly prevalent and are frequently triggered by increased oil secretion caused by our body's stress response. In addition to learning psychological skills for dealing with stress and anxiety, you might profit from utilizing BHAs like salicylic acid. This aids in breaking down excess oil seen in irritated or congested pores. Furthermore, utilizing treatments that have benzoyl peroxide is an effective strategy to combat the bacteria that trigger acne. This helps to prevent further outbreaks.

How Can I Eliminate Dark Circles Beneath My Eyes Permanently?

Dark circles are fairly prevalent and usually indicate aging and/or collagen loss in the eye region. To completely eradicate them, use a mixture of clinical and natural therapies. For instance, a gentle chemical peel that utilizes glycolic acid can help boost collagen formation and give the skin a radiant tone. At home, put a cold compress on the affected region for 10 minutes each morning and evening.

What Will Help to Tighten Your Skin?

There are a multitude of treatments and products available to assist in increasing skin elasticity and strengthening the overall surface. Aloe vera, for instance, contains malic acid, which promotes plumper and younger-looking skin. Furthermore, procedures like lymphatic massage utilize specialized equipment to enhance blood circulation in the impacted region, resulting in tighter skin. Finally, products like retinol serums provide excellent anti-aging benefits, allowing more attractive skin to develop over time.

How Do You Remove Blackheads?

Blackheads arise when extra hair and oil block an open pore. The most efficient method to eliminate blackheads is to have a high-quality face treatment. Chemical peels are an excellent example. This is because chemical peels, particularly ones containing salicylic acid, assist in exfoliating the skin and unclogging damaged pores, resulting in a cleaner, blemish-free complexion.

Is There a Do-It-Yourself Treatment for Acne Scars?

Acne scars are fairly prevalent, but fortunately, they typically need little to no treatment. But if you are experiencing severe acne or you have a strong urge to pick your spots, acne scarring, on the other hand, might be more severe. There are several treatments available to help decrease and erase acne scars and there are also things you may do to help eliminate them on your own. These include utilizing salicylic acid and lactic acid to scrub the skin. Retinol treatments are also effective at increasing skin cell renewal, which helps to prevent scarring.

Do you need to utilize toners and what are they?

One of the most perplexing skincare topics is the function of toners and whether they are required. Basically, toners are products that are utilized to eliminate excess oil, makeup and grime. In essence, toners are unnecessary, particularly if you use an excellent cleanser. This is due to the fact that they frequently trigger dryness or discomfort. However, toners, on the other hand, can help reduce the size of bigger pores, which is beneficial for individuals with oily skin type or people with acne-prone skin.

How Do I Remove Dry Skin at Home?

Dry skin is a prevalent skin problem that can be readily treated at home. All you have to do is update your skincare routine. For instance, try utilizing a natural moisturizer with no irritants. Pure aloe Vera gel is the perfect natural moisturizer. In addition, wash your face two times a day with a moderate cleanser to help remove grime and dead skin. Lastly, ensure to exfoliate once a week to eliminate extra dry skin and promote improved cell renewal.

What Acne Treatments Can Prevent Dry Skin?

People who have acne often grumble about having dry patches that follow their breakouts. Fortunately, dermoi provides the ideal solution. The Osmosis Acne Healing Treatment utilizes a 2% vitamin A infusion to repair epidermal quality and reestablish hydro-lipid balance. As an outcome, this therapy decreases unpleasant irritation and gives you a clearer, brighter skin tone.

Is it safer to utilize vitamin C serum in the morning or evening?

Vitamin C serums provide numerous benefits when used in both your morning and nighttime skincare regimen. Applying a vitamin C serum in your morning skincare regimen improves your skin's ability to neutralize damaging free radicals. These can accumulate during the day and degrade essential skin collagen. On the contrary, by including vitamin C serums in your nighttime regimen, you can reduce your chance of dangerous photosensitivity. This is given that vitamin C can increase skin sensitivity to sunshine.

How Do You Prevent Skin Aging?

Sadly, aging skin is a natural aspect of growing older, but there are certain things you can do to help keep your skin from aging too quickly. First and foremost, use sunscreen every day to shield your skin from severe sun damage. Sun damage can result in the creation of wrinkles and dark patches. It is also suggested that you use mild cleansers to prevent excessive dryness or itchiness, which can lead to skin inflammation. Collagen supplements, like Skinade, are another effective strategy to prevent skin aging. Collagen production falls by 1% every year as we age. As an outcome, this triggers the signs of aging, such as dryness, drooping skin, wrinkles and dullness. Collagen supplements counteract and prevent these effects.

When Should I Start Applying Anti-Aging Skincare Products?

This is one of the most commonly asked skincare questions. Many professionals recommend that you start applying anti-aging products in your twenties and keep adding them as part of your daily skincare regimen. This is because your skin stops manufacturing collagen in your twenties. As a result, anti-aging products provide prophylactic strategies against apparent indicators of aging.

How can I eliminate hormonal acne?

This is one of the most prevalent skincare questions. When it pertains to hormonal acne, a multifaceted strategy is required. The greatest solution consists of a series of measures targeted at regulating the hormonal background. This strategy entails using appropriate skincare products, adhering to a balanced diet and treating existing physical issues.

Can stress trigger acne?

This is also one of the commonly asked skincare questions. Yes, stress can have an indirect effect on the appearance of acne. In general, being stressed affects your physical and physiological status. As a result, acne and breakouts might show up.

Which vitamins are best for beautiful skin?

When it comes to prevalent skin health questions, this one is very relevant. To keep the skin healthy and attractive, it is critical to nourish cells with important nutrients. Vitamins C, B and E are vital because they have antioxidant qualities and improve the protective barrier. Moreover, other nutrients are necessary. Zinc, collagen, Omega fatty acids and selenium are a few examples.

What skincare ingredients should I avoid during pregnancy?

Pregnant ladies often contemplate such skincare questions and solutions. For them, it's crucial to avoid salicylic acid, retinoids and certain essential oils. Pregnant women should avoid cosmetics that have formaldehyde, aluminum chloride, phthalates, tetracycline, dihydroxyacetone, thioglycolic acid, benzoyl peroxide hydroquinone, parabens and oxybenzone.

Is it dangerous to use alcohol on the skin?

Definitely. Alcohol-containing skincare products should be avoided because they dry out the skin. While most individuals need to moisturize their cells to keep them hydrated, alcohol also has a reverse effect.

What products do I require for a basic yet efficient skincare routine?

A simple and efficient skincare routine requires products like a face cleanser, toner, moisturizer, body cream and sunscreen.

Which ingredients should I search for in a moisturizer?

The components to search for in a moisturizer involve niacinamide (a kind of vitamin B3), glycerin, kojic acid, etc. Some of these components have been shown to mitigate skin problems such as acne, hyperpigmentation and skin dullness while enhancing hydration.

What is the difference between AHA and BHA?

AHAs and BHAs are both chemical exfoliants; however, the ways they work differ. AHAs (alpha hydroxy acids) are water-soluble and exfoliate the outer layer of skin, whilst BHAs (beta hydroxy acids) can reach further into the pores to eliminate oil, grime and dead skin cells. Similarly, AHAs are excellent for enhancing skin texture and lowering the formation of fine lines and wrinkles, but BHAs are particularly good for those with acne-prone or oily skin. Illustrations of AHAs comprise lactic acid, mandelic acid and glycolic acid. Illustration of BHAs comprise salicylic acid and tropic acid.

What security measures should I take when utilizing AHA and BHA?

When utilizing AHA or BHA, do not rub them on open cuts or sunburned regions. Similarly, remember to utilize a moisturizer and sunscreen after rubbing these components to protect your skin because they can dry out and render you more sensitive to the sun. Just use these products two to three times per week, at night, as excessive use can irritate your skin.

Bottom line: if you happen to have sensitive skin, it's ideal to see a skincare specialist before incorporating these components into your skincare regimen. They can help you decide whether these acids are suitable for you and which to apply.

Do you need a serum in your skincare regimen?

Serums are an important part of any skincare routine, but they are not necessary for everybody. They are formulated with concentrated components that address certain skin issues. A vitamin C serum, for instance, can assist in lightening your skin and reducing dark spots. Hyaluronic acid serums moisturize the skin, whilst azelaic acid and retinol serums can aid in fighting acne and hyperpigmentation. In a similar way, collagen serums help diminish fine lines and wrinkles. So, if you have particular skin issues, incorporating a serum into your daily routine can be an absolute game changer.

How long should you wait before using skincare products?

When stacking up your skincare products, it's ideal to allow two to three minutes for each one to absorb before adding the next. However, the amount of time required depends on the product's thickness and contents.

Is it okay to blend vitamin C oil, Niacinamide and collagen serum and then apply them to the face?

Serums should be applied separately at least two to five minutes apart. If you happen to have sensitive skin, avoid using vitamin C serum and niacinamide serum together. We suggest applying vitamin C in the morning routine and Niacinamide in the nighttime routine or vice versa.

What is the best technique to treat sensitive skin?

Be cautious with it! Constantly wash sensitive skin carefully and avoid abrasive cleaners. Avoid products containing unpleasant ingredients. Rather, look for products that are specially labeled for sensitive skin.

How can I correct an uneven skin tone?

An uneven complexion is created from an uneven dispersion of pigment. Sun exposure and hormonal fluctuations may also contribute to this problem. Some serums, lotions and moisturizers, particularly those containing vitamin C, can assist in balancing out your complexion. It is also feasible that your skin will develop an uneven tone as a result of the accumulation of dead skin cells. If this is the case, exfoliating once a day or every two days might help balance out your skin tone.

What's the distinction between a day spa and a medical spa?

There are numerous therapies available at either a day spa or a med spa. A med spa may address more challenging skin conditions and its providers typically have experience with and are licensed to undertake medical aesthetic operations. Another distinction between the two is that therapies at a med spa are overseen by a medical practitioner.

How long till I begin to see results?

Results can differ based on the person and the products being used. The consistency with which you follow your skincare regimen is crucial to the effectiveness of your results. Thus, we recommend three to six months for the skin to improve from bad to good. Results might appear sooner than this starting point.

At what age should I begin anti-aging treatments?

When it pertains to anti-aging products, particularly those containing antioxidants, the conventional recommendation is to begin in your early twenties. Taking preventative measures in your twenties will keep your skin appearing youthful in the long term.

I have dark skin; should I apply sunscreen?

Darker skin produces more melanin, but this only provides a limited level of protection. Dark skin might become sunburned and develop skin cancer. A good Ultraviolet sunscreen is essential for all skin types.

What's the distinction between an esthetician and a dermatologist?

A dermatologist undergoes medical school and may have twelve to fourteen years of postgraduate education. Aestheticians are specially trained to concentrate on skincare and offering non-invasive procedures.

What skincare products are effective with chemotherapy?

The greatest products to utilize will soothe and hydrate your skin. Skin creams that include antioxidants to replenish while suppressing moisture loss can be quite beneficial.

Where do skin tags come from?

Skin tags typically grow in the folds of your skin. There is no conclusive reason known for their development, but it is considered to be caused by skin friction.

Can I use lime and lemon on my skin?

Lemons and limes have components that are used in several cosmetic treatments; nonetheless, there has been an upsurge in the misuse of these fruits in topical applications. We do not recommend utilizing skincare products that are not regulated by regulatory agencies on your skin.

Prior to using a product on the skin, it's ideal to conduct a patch test. You also have to rule out any allergic reactions. We urge that you speak with your provider, who may give recommendations for safe skin care products to utilize on your skin.

About the Author

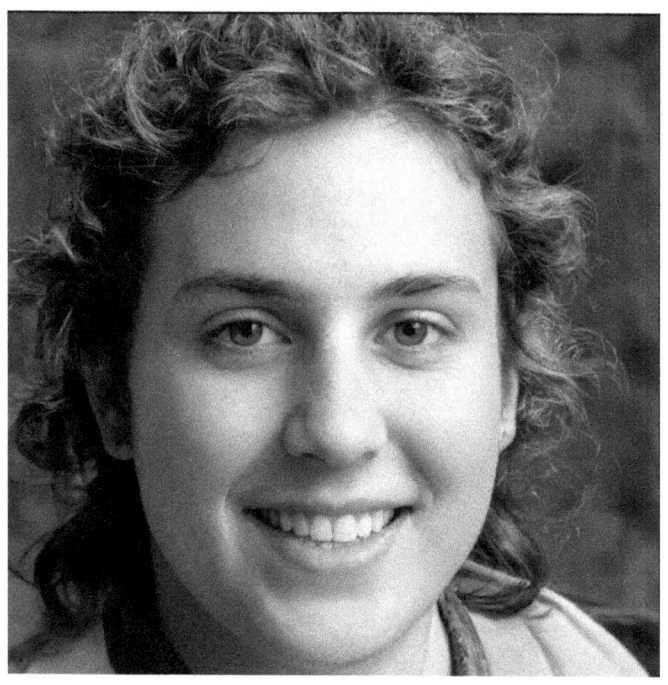

Whitney F. Bowe is a passionate skincare enthusiast and wellness writer with a deep commitment to helping others achieve healthy, glowing skin. With years of research and personal exploration into skincare routines, ingredients, and holistic beauty practices, Whitney brings a relatable and practical voice to the world of skincare education.

Her work focuses on making skincare approachable for everyone—no jargon, no overwhelm, just honest advice backed by science and experience. When she's not writing, Whitney enjoys testing new skincare products, experimenting with DIY treatments, and connecting with readers who share her love for self-care and confidence through skin health.

This is her debut guide, written with the goal of empowering readers to make informed choices and build routines that work for their unique skin types and lifestyles.

www.ingramcontent.com/pod-product-compliance
Lightning Source LLC
Chambersburg PA
CBHW051542020426
42333CB00016B/2056